Second Chance

A Sister's Act of Love

DR. M. P. RAVINDRA NATHAN

AUTHOR OF "STORIES FROM MY HEART"

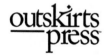

Dedicated to my dear *Kochopol,*
Mrs: Ratnam Sivaraman
I am truly blessed to be your brother

A beautiful soul loves without condition,
Talks without bad intention,
Gives without a reason and most of all
Cares for people without any expectations

Anonymous

SECOND CHANCE
A SISTER'S ACT OF LOVE

After undergoing a kidney transplant surgery in a Minneapolis hospital, I was lying in the intensive care unit, floating between anesthesia-induced fog and periods of lucidity. The pain and swelling in the belly at the site of the operation were mounting. Unbeknownst to me, I was developing major complications. I could sense the nurses and doctors running around frantically shouting orders to each other,

"Take him back to the O.R. this second!"

"Get an ultrasound of the femoral artery"

"He may be developing a major clot"

"Oh! He is losing blood pressure!"

That was the time I prayed hard, "God, I need you now!"

As I slipped into unconsciousness, I felt the presence of something supernatural.

Did I see the angelic face of my own father who has been gone for twenty years, coming to rescue me as I lay at the precipice between life and death?

Did he sit by my bedside and gently stroke my belly and smile at me?

Did he say in a comforting voice, "Ravi, don't worry, you have a decidedly unfinished life, you can't go now?"

I knew right then I would make it through this ordeal and live to tell my story.

And here is my story.........

M. P. RAVINDRA NATHAN

TABLE OF CONTENTS

FOREWORD

SECOND CHANCE
A SISTER'S ACT OF LOVE

In this touching, inspiring and true story of survival, Dr. Ravindra Nathan recounts his own experience after fate hands him a challenge resulting in the need for a kidney transplant. Through his eyes and words, we learn the functions of this vital organ, the imminent necessity for someone else's kidney to allow survival with a reasonable quality of life, and the ultimate loving sacrifice of a sister that miraculously infused a second, productive life into him.

Readers will be inspired by the dynamics of a loving family which is reflected through all his recurring ordeals as well as the gracious support from his immediate and extended family, friends and the medical community of which he is part.

With great nerve and verve, the author details the experience of the complications after surgery, and without any self-pity or show of regret, tells us of the tribulations he had to go through in the following years, as a person on medications to sustain and protect his newly gifted organ. After every fall, he got up and fought his way through a series of calamitous health crises to come out victorious, now having completed over twenty-three years post-transplant. At the same time, the smiling face in the follow up-photographs reflects his gratitude to his devoted wife, the people who took care of him and to The Almighty.

The reader will experience the joy of blessings received, and learn a road-map as to how to handle life's misfortunes gracefully until the light shines through for a glorious future. We wish for you a second chance if you need one, as was given to Ravindra Nathan.

Shakuntala Rajagopal, MD
Physician and Author of
"Song of the Mountains," "Radha" and "*My Pilgrimage to Maa Ganga*"

INTRODUCTION

About three decades ago, I got the shock of my life. I developed an incurable kidney disease called IgA Nephropathy, a disease that will inexorably progress to kidney failure, necessitating a kidney transplant. Interestingly this would also be the very first surgery on my body and I was beset with one complication after another. Often, I was in abysmal depths of anxiety not knowing what the future held for me. Fortunately with the help of my family, primarily my sister who donated one of her kidneys to me, and my wife who attended to me every step of the way plus a group of good doctors and friends, I survived all the crises and achieved some stability in life. My eventual recovery from a serious illness after going through a complicated course is a true testament to the miracle of modern medicine. Twenty-four years have passed since my kidney transplant and I continue to be active, loving every moment of life.

The main reason I wrote this book is to let the readers know – both lay public and medical personnel – that a kidney transplant is the best treatment for kidney failure and, even if you encounter complications during or after surgery, with proper management you can recover and live to enjoy your life for many years, as I have. My unique story takes you through the details of how kidney failure could happen to anybody, even to someone who is apparently in good health, the complicated surgery and recovery process I experienced, multiple other medical crises, the difficult journey of my sister, the donor, to come to USA, the ground work of the transplant coordinators and more. Being a physician and a practicing cardiologist familiar with the inner workings of the body and preventive care, you might think that I would have been an unlikely candidate for kidney failure. But *dis-ease* can happen to anyone; yes, even doctors can become seriously ill, necessitating such surgeries as an organ transplant. Anybody who is facing the challenge of a kidney or any other organ transplant, needs to be familiar and comfortable with what's involved in the preparation—from getting a matching donor (cadaveric or live), to undergoing the surgery, and through the sometimes complicated recovery process that follows. Then there will be frequent blood tests, doctor visits, drug adjustments and lifestyle changes with which to comply.

Transplantation as a science has evolved significantly and the surgery for both the donor and recipient have become a lot easier now compared to when I had it over twenty-three years ago. Donor nephrectomy (removal of kidney) can be done through minimally invasive 'laparoscopic' or keyhole surgery with robotic-assisted technology wherein a kidney can be removed easily through tiny incisions on the side of the abdomen. This makes the hospital recovery time far shorter for the kidney donor. The same thing is applicable to transplant recipients as well. It's my hope that this book will be a useful companion for any and all patients suffering from chronic kidney disease, their caretakers, the treating physicians, and other medical and nursing staff involved in their care as well as for the general public. As the national organ shortage continues, living related or unrelated matching donors may be the best solution, better than cadaveric transplants. New immunologic treatments are being developed that will facilitate transplantation with even an unmatched organ from an incompatible live donor. That will be a great encouragement for all patients waiting for transplants and indeed, a big step up for science. And hopefully, altruism among the public is prevalent now as we are beginning to hear stories about total strangers coming forward to donate one of their precious organs to save a life. At the end of the book, I have included some general instructions on how to become an organ donor and how to maintain or protect the function of your native kidneys as well as that of the transplanted kidney.

Ultimately, we need to trust our own body—its beauty, resiliency and ability for recovery, no matter how ravaged it is with disease processes. I hope you enjoy this book and find inspiration from my story. It begins in 1989, which seems like a long time ago but the beauty of this book is that I am still alive and continue to enjoy my life with a functioning transplanted kidney as I write it in 2018.

M. P. Ravindra Nathan MD

PROLOGUE

March 18, 1994 - Brooksville, Florida

The phone rang. Almost instinctively I knew this must be the call from my older sister, Ratnam, in India. For a couple of days now, I'd been waiting for this call.

"Daddy, this is Ratna *Chitta* (aunt), pick up the phone quickly. She must have gotten her visa!" Sandra, my daughter, called from upstairs. There was palpable excitement in her voice. A senior at Hernando High, Sandra (we call her Sanu) was preparing for her final semester exams. I was in the kitchen downstairs preparing a simple breakfast.

With tremulous hands, I picked up the telephone while silently reciting a prayer to Lord *Ganesha*, the remover of all obstacles. I knew my time was running out. God, please don't let me down now, I kept mumbling.

"Ravi, is that you?" Ratnam's voice came through clearly, covering ten thousand transatlantic miles from Chennai to Brooksville. There was no static, no interruption.

"Yes, *Kochoppol*, this is me, Ravi. Tell me the good news," I said. I always addressed her as *Kochoppol*, which meant "youngest of my three older sisters."

"I'm sorry, Ravi," Ratnam said, her voice cracking. I could almost see tears flowing down her cheeks, as she struggled to complete the sentence. "Both Thankamani (our younger sister) and myself were refused visa by the American Consulate in Chennai. I shall write all the details to you. The Consulate staff was unhelpful, plain inconsiderate. I am calling you from a public phone booth."

Then silence. The phone went dead.

I felt dizzy and my head started reeling. Suddenly, darkness spread rapidly from one corner of the room engulfing me quickly. First I thought the whole thing was a bad dream. But soon I realized what I heard was real.

How could this be? My kidney failure had progressed to the point that I would have to start dialysis soon unless I got a kidney transplant. Both my sisters shared my blood group, so they would be my best chance for a donor. And they were prepared to come to the U.S. for tissue typing and matching tests as well as other work-up needed before being considered for kidney donation. I had sent all the necessary certificates and affidavits, including the two required letters from the transplant nephrologists attending me. What more could they possibly want?

Now what! I was stumped for an answer. Hooked up to a dialysis machine three times a week? And frequent hospitalizations? Unable to travel anywhere? What kind of life would that be? I had heard several grim stories from some of my patients about their experience on dialysis.

"My life changed the day I was put on dialysis," said Roger, whom I had followed for some time in my clinic. He had chronic heart disease and end-stage kidney disease. Although some of his symptoms had improved on dialysis, his life had changed dramatically because of the time commitment dialysis required and the fatigue he felt afterwards. Getting around was difficult too. "Now I have to arrange with a dialysis unit wherever I travel, way ahead of time and then get my own transportation to the dialysis center where I am staying," he told me. "I'm so afraid to stay in a hotel for fear of any emergencies that might crop up at night. The only time I go out of town now is to Washington, D.C., where my daughter lives; she makes all the arrangements. For the rest of my life, I am more or less stuck here. And going abroad is out of question, maybe up to Canada at the most, but nowhere else," he added in desperation.

I dreaded even the thought of dialysis for myself. I liked working with patients and wanted to continue my practice of cardiology, the love of my life. And I enjoyed going to the hospital, taking care of acute emergencies like heart attacks and cardiac arrhythmias, inserting pacemakers in the middle of the night and saving patients' lives. I was always in my element when dealing with the challenges in the intensive and coronary care units of my hospitals. Just the thought that I could make a difference in their lives was a big motivator and filled me with pride and purpose in life. Would I have to give up all this?

I had just turned fifty-three and there was plenty of life left in me. But I didn't know what I would do if I had to stop working. With dialysis looming in my immediate future, I felt like my life was closing in on me. My eyes pooled with tears. I couldn't speak.

Did she really say she didn't get the visa?

PART I
THE STORM

1

A MEMORABLE TRIP

January 1989, New York

I BOARDED A flight from J.F.K. airport, New York, to Mumbai (previously Bombay). This was the first time I would travel without my wife Susheela. I felt a little lonely and uncomfortable although still excited about going home to Kerala, the southernmost state in India. I would be attending two weddings there, the primary purpose of this visit, within a tight schedule of just two weeks.

My two nieces, Maya and Indu, were getting married and this gave me an opportunity to see all my folks. Usually, Susheela and I take our vacation during the summer months with our school-going children. In addition, winter in Florida is quite busy for doctors when the seasonal residents from up north, the 'snowbirds,' return to their winter homes. But this trip in January was an exciting opportunity I couldn't pass up. Weddings are always a time for family reunions and fellowship and I had always enjoyed bonding with my kith and kin.

The Air India jumbo jet with the fancy name, *Emperor Ashoka,* was crowded. That wasn't unusual, with the bargain rates for the to and fro trips. I liked the spicy Indian dishes they served and the melodious in flight music on seven different channels. A turbaned sentry welcomed passengers with a *namaste* at the waiting lounge and another one at the door of this "floating palace in the air," a royal welcome, indeed! They screened three movies during the trip. There were plenty of demanding passengers and screaming children, part and parcel of an Indian's travel entourage. But the 'air hostesses' (flight attendants) in their colorful *saris* and sweet smiles always handled them adeptly. I took it all in stride since this was my tenth trip to India after coming to USA in 1972.

The flight was not without some unexpected excitement. As we crossed the Irish Sea toward Heathrow Airport, London, one gentleman suddenly developed chest pain.

"Are there any physicians onboard?" an announcement came from the overhead speakers.

My right hand went up immediately and I was promptly escorted to one of the front seats. The air hostess, relieved to see at least one doctor on board to serve in a crisis, checked my credentials, and satisfied, asked me where I practiced.

"In Brooksville, Florida," I said. "I am a cardiologist."

"That's great!" she exclaimed, rushing me to the patient. The gentleman, about seventy, was a little pale and sweaty. His blood pressure (BP) was up. Careful auscultation of the heart revealed abnormal heart sounds including a third sound or S3 gallop, usually an indication of some strain on the heart in an older patient. Brief questioning revealed that he suffered from *angina pectoris* that often manifests as chest pain or discomfort—a tell-tale sign of coronary heart disease.

I hoped he was not developing an acute heart attack since it would be difficult to give any effective treatment at 35,000 feet up in the air. I promptly got him to lie down on the three seats in that row and gave him a sublingual nitroglycerine pill that I always carried in my tote bag along with a few other medical paraphernalia, handy for such emergencies. The captain brought a small cylinder of oxygen, and he was started on two liters per minute through a nasal cannula. He was not a diabetic, so hypoglycemia or low blood sugar was unlikely. But I decided it wouldn't hurt to give him some IV glucose to perk him up.

The next step was to get an EKG (electrocardiogram). Unfortunately, the plane had only an older model, single strip EKG machine that spat out a continuous recording of just one lead from the electrode placed on the chest, so I couldn't get a standard 12 lead EKG. The strip showed regular sinus rhythm with frequent extra beats called ventricular ectopics, which further strengthened my belief that he was likely having true angina and might even be developing a heart attack. The plane soon landed in Heathrow and the paramedics, radioed earlier and waiting at the terminal, immediately entered the plane with a stretcher. "Okay, we'll take it from here," they said, authoritatively.

"Can we do a full twelve lead EKG quickly?" I asked. "Then we can inform the receiving hospital what to expect."

They looked at me quizzically. "Who are you?" they asked and wanted to see my credentials.

"I am a board-certified cardiologist practicing in Florida," I answered confidently.

"We are taking him to the local hospital where they will do all the necessary tests. He doesn't need an EKG now," one of the paramedics said emphatically and they whisked him away. Well, so much for courtesy!

The rest of my trip was uneventful until we landed in Mumbai. One of the busiest airports in the world, it was teeming with people. I negotiated my way through the crowd with some difficulty and collected my baggage, two large suitcases swollen with lots of goodies for my family members, many of them anticipating a gift from their uncle in USA.

Going through the Indian customs at Mumbai was always a harrowing experience. Even though I had opted to go through the green channel meant for those not carrying any illegal or dutiable items to declare, the customs officer decided to check everything inside the boxes. I knew they were specifically looking for electronic gadgets like calculators, portable tape recorders, (CD players were not available at that time), cameras or gold. Then he dipped into the open suitcase and picked up a fancy flashlight and a Parker pen for himself before waving his hand dismissively, indicating "Okay, you may go now."

Once outside, I was promptly greeted by *Damummavan,* Susheela's uncle settled in Mumbai, with his son, Jayan, a dashing young man who knew his way around the big metropolis. I was quickly taken to their nice flat in Khar where a hot, delectable breakfast was waiting cooked by *Damummavan's* wife whom we called *Ammayi (aunty).*

That afternoon, I caught a flight to Kochi, the largest city in Kerala. National Geographic once described Kerala as 'God's own country' because of its rich heritage, lush greenery, numerous lakes, rivers and backwaters, high level of education, religious tolerance and amiable people. Soon, the plane landed in Wellington Island Naval Airport in Kochi, only twenty miles from the village where I grew up. As soon as I walked into the arrival building, a chorus of warm welcome arose from the cheering crowd, my family members and friends, all eagerly waiting for over an hour to receive me. It gave me goose bumps.

January 1989

Going home has always been a wonderful experience. I was born in a village called Njarakkal, which is part of a small island, Vypin in Kerala. About fifteen miles long and three to four miles wide, Vypin is densely populated; many of the locals are fishermen, small shopkeepers and daily wage earners. I could see a lot of changes on my island. What used to be desolate roads with hardly any vehicles had turned into busy thoroughfares with a cavalcade of mixed sorts – cars, buses, three-wheeler auto-rickshaws, bullock carts and hand-drawn carriages. Several new shopping centers and hospitals had risen up.

Finally, I reached my ancestral house, now occupied by my older sister and her family, to a rousing reception. It was a thrilling occasion, a homecoming filled with joy and satisfaction. I choked up on hearing the familiar sound of the holy conch being blown from the nearby ancient temple, a relic from my childhood; I was certainly home! The fact that just a couple of days ago, I was in the middle of a frenzied professional life, trying to balance hospital and clinic work with a domestic life, was soon forgotten.

~~~

Both the wedding ceremonies went very well—Maya's in Trissur in a special wedding auditorium, and Indu's at the famous Guruvayur Temple in Kerala. Later I attended one more wedding of a friend's daughter. I participated in all the delightful ceremonies to my heart's content.

What comes after an Indian Hindu wedding ceremony is one of the most exciting vegetarian gastronomic delights. It is a twenty course feast, *sadhya,* a highly-sophisticated cuisine with the inspired use of spices and an added touch of sweetness in selected preparations, with desserts galore.

The only problem with these gourmet feasts is their salt, spice and fat content. In America, I am accustomed to a less spicy low fat diet, so my stomach acts up whenever I travel anywhere in India. Recently, my blood pressure (BP) had started edging upwards, so I had been on a low-salt diet too. But once in India, I was constantly invited to my relatives' homes where they fed me delicious foods that included spicy curries, salt-laden pickles, snacks and more. So far, during this trip, I had fully enjoyed all three of the feasts.

I think that almost did me in!

One night I woke up with a pounding headache. The severe throbbing around my forehead was almost unbearable. This caught me by surprise since I almost never get headaches even under stress from dealing with complex problems in the ICU (intensive care unit) or handling difficult situations on the home front. But now my pulse was full and bounding; I felt flushed and restless. I knew right away something was wrong; this was definitely not my usual self.

Had my BP gone up? I checked it with a portable BP machine that I usually carried during these long trips and to my dismay, found it had jumped to 180/116 (normal being around 120/80)! A repeat measurement showed the same numbers. The sudden realization that I had developed significant hypertension (high blood pressure) all of a sudden hit me like a fist in the face. I was totally clueless. I took one pill of the medicine *Vasotec* (enalapril) that I had brought for a hypertensive relative, hoping to get some relief from the headaches. In a few minutes, my BP was down to 150/90, and I felt better. One more pill brought it further down, so I decided to put myself on a two-pill-a-day regime.

The local general practitioner, a family friend, came around later to check me and she also confirmed that I had developed hypertension. My hectic work load and the stress it generated coupled with recent indulgence in salty diet may have contributed to this. I made a mental note to relax more and be careful what I ate and continue my exercise routine. Hopefully my BP would be controlled with just a little medication and I should be back to normal soon. I remembered the two plaques hanging in my study given by my friends who had seen my super busy schedules and stressful life.

"Don't take life too seriously," said one.

"Don't fret over small things. And everything in life is small," the other one read.

Well, that was exactly what I was going to do. But I couldn't shake the feeling that something was seriously wrong with my body. I was very eager to get back to Florida and have a full work up.

I had no idea that my life was about to change forever.

2

A Disturbing Diagnosis

February, 1989

A LONG TRANSATLANTIC flight brought me back to New York and I immediately felt better; I was back in the U.S., my home turf. With customs and other formalities quickly over, I caught the flight to Tampa and then drove to Brooksville.

For the past nine years, Brooksville, a small, historic town in Hernando County, established by the Spanish conqueror Hernando De Soto, had been my home in the USA. Located in Central Florida, it is primarily a residential community of some 70,000 people (It is now up to 180,000 as of 2018). Our only claim to fame is the presence of 'Weeki Wachee Springs,' a Florida attraction featuring mermaids and beautifully choreographed underwater shows. I had become very fond of this rural place and always felt right at home here. We do get frequent visitors from up north who come here to enjoy the many attractions and tourist spots like Busch Gardens (Tampa), Kennedy Space Center (Cape

Canaveral), Disney World (Orlando) or the fabulous beaches—all just a short distance away.

The day after I landed, I went to Brooksville Regional Hospital where I practice, to have a few preliminary tests. The results of the detailed blood workup and urinalysis caught me by surprise. My urine showed lots of albumin (a protein in the blood) or *albuminuria*, an indication of kidney damage. The serum electrolytes were markedly off too. Two major indices, blood urea nitrogen (BUN) and serum *creatinine*, were elevated to 55 and 2.2, the normal levels being <24 and <1.3 respectively. Serum *creatinine* (Cr), a blood test, is a pretty accurate measure of kidney function and an increased level indicates the presence of kidney damage. The last time those numbers were checked was several years ago while I worked at the New Jersey College of Medicine, Newark, when all blood work was completely normal.

My worst fears were coming true. Just as I had suspected, there was something seriously wrong with me. The sudden surge in blood pressure was only the tip of the iceberg. For further confirmation, I did a special test called 'creatinine clearance' (which measures the amount of creatinine in a 24 hour urine specimen and helps to estimate the *glomerular filtration rate* or GFR, an important measure of kidney function), that also turned out to be abnormal, down to 51 cc/ minute (Normal range for a male being 90 -130 ml per minute). Now I had to consult a nephrologist (kidney specialist), pronto!

One concern I had was that my illness would become public knowledge if I saw a local physician to manage my care or used local labs for frequent blood tests. Brooksville was a small town where everyone knew everyone else and keeping a secret was difficult. The medical community was small and all physicians knew each other well. Although my physicians would be discrete with personal matters of a colleague, I couldn't be certain about trusting the ancillary staff to keep my illness a secret. Therefore, I decided to go to the Watson Clinic in Lakeland, Florida, a reputed regional referral center only fifty five miles away, for further evaluation, thinking that a consult with a senior *nephrologist* (kidney specialist) there would be the best option. Interestingly, I still felt quite healthy and physically fit and looked normal in every respect, my close friends would say. In spite of the abnormal blood tests, I had no problem maintaining my exercise routine that included gentle jogging three miles twice a week and a couple of sessions of tennis. And I continued my cardiovascular practice without interruption.

Dr. Mark Stampfel, the staff *nephrologist* at Watson Clinic, was cordial and listened to my story patiently. He noted my history of allergies. I was a bit anxious, so my blood pressure had gone up while waiting in his office. After a thorough physical examination, my urine sample was examined. There was a lot of protein and some blood in the urine; the sediment showed granular and red blood cell casts, clear signs of kidney damage.

"Well, you certainly have hypertension and the picture is compatible with a *glomerulopathy*," he said impassively.

That meant I had some kind of inflammation of the *glomeruli*, which are clusters of small blood vessels inside each *nephron*, the basic functional unit in the kidney that filter waste products and excess water from the blood. Both my kidneys had sustained some damage, and it was likely it would worsen slowly and eventually lead to kidney failure.

"What do you think is the cause?" I pressed him for an answer. I couldn't believe this was all secondary to my high blood pressure. Chronic kidney damage usually occurs with long-standing hypertension, but my hypertension manifested itself only in the past month and I didn't have diabetes, so how the kidneys could be damaged so quickly?

"We will have to do a renal biopsy." His answer was terse, not wanting to venture a diagnosis at this time.

Thoroughly rattled, I shuddered at the thought of someone sticking a long needle into my back and taking a piece of my kidney. During my medical residency in the early 70s, I had seen enough complications like heavy bleeding, including some requiring surgery. One particular memory still lingered in my mind. The renal fellow attempted to do a kidney biopsy. He placed a grill on the patient's back around the kidney area, took X-rays to locate the position of the kidney in relation to the grill, and assessed the depth of the kidney from the surface to determine how far the needle should go inside the abdomen, as was the usual practice. Ultrasound guidance was not available in those days. The needle was inserted and directed toward the kidney to get a sliver of the tissue. He had to pass the needle a couple of times before getting a sample which was promptly sent to the pathology department for microscopic examination.

The pathologist called back shortly afterwards and said sarcastically to the fellow, "What did you send me? *shish kebob?* There is a piece of liver and a tiny piece of kidney here, back to back. *Make sure he is not bleeding from the liver!*" It was clear that the needle had pierced the edge of the liver before it entered the kidney. Fortunately, the patient recovered without any major complications, but it had left an indelible impression in my mind about what could go wrong during a kidney biopsy if not done properly. The radiologist in my small hospital did a few of them periodically without any complications, though.

"Do I really need a biopsy?" I asked Dr. Stampfl worriedly, sounding like an apprehensive lay person, not a physician.

"We do it under ultrasound guidance now," he explained. "Complications are rare but bleeding can occur at times. We will have a couple of units of blood ready for transfusion," he added, encouragingly, and proceeded to schedule a date for the biopsy.

All of a sudden, I felt very depressed. How quickly does one's life change! Just a few days ago, I was a happy man, working twelve hours a day and still exercising and enjoying the remaining hours. At hospital meetings, when we were often treated to rich and tasty filet mignons and delicious desserts like cheesecakes or pineapple truffles, I was always careful to order a fruit platter and salad, eliciting a kind of admiration from my colleagues. Peggy Gangarosa, the chief of pathology would often remark: "Look at what Dr. Nathan eats! Oh my, what a stickler for healthy diet! We should all follow his example."

Well, in spite of following a strict healthy lifestyle, I was down with a serious kidney disease. The anxious doctor in me could see the prognosis clearly etched on the wall. My poor kidneys were failing, and in a few short years, I would be hooked on to a dialysis machine. Nephrologists had always told me during patient discussions and conferences that by the time the creatinine levels are up, considerable damage has already occurred to the kidneys. The rest of the normal kidney tissue would eventually follow suit and this meant, in a short time, I could be heading to the dialysis unit. That was a scary thought indeed and anxiety became my constant companion.

Susheela tried to console me and calm my nerves. "After all, this is not cancer, why are you so worried?" A petite yet strong woman and ever my pillar of support, she was always ready to face with a smile the curve balls life would throw at us. Being a pediatrician she saw plenty of sick children, some with serious illnesses including cancer. Both of us worked in the same office, a nice professional building we constructed together. Occasionally, when I glanced toward her side of the waiting room, I would see children with bald heads from chemotherapy and some with major deformities or disabilities. For many of them, the future looked bleak. But she always gave them hope, kept them good-humored and helped them in any way she could, so they could cope with their challenges.

"You make it look like this is a tragedy or something," she added. "Don't worry too much. We will get a second opinion and explore all modalities of treatment. You have always been a positive person. Do not let this illness defeat you."

Encouraging words, just what I needed to hear. But with disbelief and skepticism about the diagnosis, I consulted some of my colleagues who felt a CT (computerized tomography) scan-guided biopsy might be better than doing it under ultrasound imaging. The chances of hitting the target were higher and complications would be less. I decided to seek a second opinion at the University of Florida Shands Hospital in Gainesville which had a reputable renal program. A consultation with Dr. Don Mars, Professor of Nephrology, was scheduled.

On February 22, 1994, I arrived at Shands outpatient nephrology clinic to be examined by a team of physicians. After the preliminaries were completed, Dr. Mars joined the team to review all the tests up to that point. He concurred with Dr. Stampfl that I do have kidney disease, probably a special type called *IgA Nephropathy* that results from the deposition of a protein from the blood, an immune globulin called *IgA*, in the kidney. A biopsy of the kidney tissue is essential for clinching the diagnosis and for proper treatment; it will help to understand the future course of the disease. And we settled on a date the following week. In my heart of hearts I still refused to believe that I had any serious kidney disease.

The night before the biopsy, Susheela and I checked into the local Holiday Inn close to the medical center. And the following morning, we promptly arrived at the radiology suite at Shands Hospital. The secretary was very cordial, but had a puzzled look on her face.

"Why are you here today?" she asked, clearly surprised.

"I have an appointment for nine a.m.," I said. "They are doing a renal biopsy on me." I tried to thrust my paperwork into her hand. "Isn't my name there?" I asked nervously.

She didn't look at me directly, but shuffled some papers back and forth and called the Radiology department to speak with a CT tech. Then, looking at me sympathetically, she said,

"Our CT machine is undergoing repairs. Your procedure has been canceled. Didn't anybody call you earlier? I'm sorry you had to make an unnecessary trip." Later I learned that the CT machine would not be functional for another couple of days.

"Nobody called me. Had I known this, I wouldn't have driven ninety miles last evening and stayed in a hotel!" I said, disappointed.

There was a lot of hushed talk behind the closed door adjacent to the reception area.

"He is a doctor coming all the way from Brooksville," somebody was saying to another person.

"Why didn't they let him know?" the other person asked.

Soon one of the radiology residents came out to apologize. This was the second time my kidney biopsy had been postponed. Chagrined I decided not to go through the procedure at this center. Who knows? With my luck, the scanner might break down again, right in the middle of the procedure!

Eager to know what was eating up my kidneys, I called my brother-in-law, Dr. Venugopal (Venu), a practicing cardiologist in West Palm Beach. He immediately contacted his close friend and colleague, Dr. M. Ramachandran, an eminent nephrologist and local practitioner, who said, "Don't worry, I will arrange Ravi's (my friends call me *Ravi*) kidney biopsy in South Miami Baptist Hospital. I know the team of nephrologists there, they are excellent. They'll do it under CT guidance." That was a tremendous relief.

Susheela and I hit the road the very next day to Miami and checked into the Baptist Hospital after a five hour drive. Venu and Dr. Ramachandran had already taken care of the preliminaries. I was scheduled for the procedure the same day. The registration clerk and nurses at the admission counter were very cordial. They collected all my insurance details and put me in a wheelchair and escorted me to a holding area at the Radiology Center where I had to don the hospital gown and be ready. The atmosphere was very pleasant, making me feel at home.

In the radiology suite, a preliminary CT of the kidneys was completed. Satisfied that there were no major anatomical abnormalities or other local changes that would affect the smooth passage of the needle, Dr. Raul De Velasco, the Chief Nephrologist, went ahead with the procedure. The skin and subcutaneous tissues were anesthetized with *lidocaine*. The right kidney was properly visualized under CT and the doctor introduced the biopsy needle gently, then withdrew and got a specimen. He changed the position slightly and did a few more passes for more tissue samples. They were all emptied into a small bottle filled with preservatives and quickly transported to the pathology lab. The biopsy specimen was processed the same day, sections made and the slides, appropriately stained and readied to be viewed under a microscope. They were sent to Dr. Victor Pardo of the University of Miami, a very reputed *immunopathologist*, for interpretation. Now we waited for the results, sweating bullets. The passage of time seemed agonizingly slow.

The verdict came the following day which blindsided me, although it shouldn't have. Yes, there was definitely damage to the kidneys. I did indeed have *IgA Nephropathy!* Although not much advanced, it wasn't mild either. Sooner or later, I was destined to go into renal failure which, of course, meant going on dialysis. Somehow, I couldn't reconcile to the cold reality. My head started buzzing with questions:

What is "IgA Nephropathy"?
How do you get it?
What did I do wrong?
Is there any way I can arrest this disease?
How long would it be before I go into full-blown renal failure?

Renal failure! Dialysis! I cringed at the thought of all that dialysis entailed. I couldn't imagine having an arterio-venous shunt in my arm, being hooked to a dialysis machine three times a week, and going through all those complications that commonly follow these procedures. Every day I saw patients, some from my own practice, admitted from the dialysis unit to the intensive care unit (ICU) because of low blood pressure or altered mental status related to volume changes in the body or some metabolic abnormalities.

I still felt healthy and continued my regular work and exercise routines, enjoying every minute of it. But for my hypertension, which

SECOND CHANCE

was under control, I didn't have any clinical signs of the disease. As the chairman of the Critical Care Committee at Brooksville Regional Hospital, I conducted the meetings well, supervised the ICU and CCU (Intensive and Coronary Care Units) and took care of my administrative as well as clinical duties in the hospital without fail.

The thought that I might have to give up all these in the near future filled me with exasperation and dismay. That scenario seemed surreal. I couldn't believe my life was coming apart at the seams in such rapid sequence. I had high hopes of doing a lot more in my life, but how long would my sick kidneys last?

"Well, nobody can say for sure," Dr. De Velasco would say later. "I know of some patients who have gone on for more than ten years after the diagnosis." He was trying to give me hope and encouragement although that still didn't pacify me. I would also have given more or less the same answer to my patients suffering from an incurable heart disease, like, "With proper treatment and precautions, you could live long."

Somehow, the future looked very uncertain and ominous, as chilly clarity set in.

3

HOW DOES ONE GET
IGA NEPHROPATHY?

March, 1989

SOME KNOWLEDGE OF the anatomy and physiology of our kidneys will be helpful to understand this disease. We don't often give enough credit to the kidneys for the amount of work they do to keep our bodies healthy. We have two kidneys, one on each side, situated in the back of the abdomen behind the peritoneal cavity, shaped like large red kidney beans. Each one has an outer cortex and inner medulla. The cortex contains millions of micro-filters called *glomeruli* which are clumps of tiny blood vessels called capillaries within the kidneys that remove waste products and excess fluids from the body and help with electrolyte balance in the blood. The excess fluid removed is sent to the bladder as urine (see Figure 1).

As blood passes through healthy kidneys, the glomeruli filter out the waste products – nitrogenous wastes from protein catabolism like urea and creatinine, uric acid from nucleic acid metabolism as well as excess water but allow the blood to retain cells and proteins the body needs. No more than a trace of protein (albumin) is found in a healthy person's urine. However, in patients with nephropathy, the damaged glomeruli allow the albumin to leak constantly into the urine (albuminuria) in large quantities. Measured over a 24-hour period, the total albumin lost in urine can exceed three grams. This is more than twenty times the amount that healthy glomeruli will allow.

In order to understand the new enemy that had invaded my body, I dug into the medical literature like research publications and text book chapters, for the latest details of this condition. Some of my nephrology colleagues sent me a number of medical reports on the disease. After reading all these, one thing became clear, my kidneys had already sustained significant damage (*nephropathy*) as shown by the large amount of protein in the urine, low albumin and high cholesterol levels in the blood, and fluid retention in the body which showed up as edema of my feet and ankles. This conglomeration of symptoms goes by the name *nephrotic syndrome.*

What exactly is IgA Nephropathy? That was the question bugging me ever since the kidney biopsy. Here is a condensed version of the scientific information about the disease.

'Immunoglobulin A Nephropathy (IgA N)' was first described by the French nephrologist, Dr. Jean Berger in 1968, hence it is often referred as Berger's disease. The disease occurs when an antibody called immunoglobulin A (IgA) gets deposited in your kidneys, causing structural damage leading to loss of kidney function.

Antibodies are essentially a type of proteins called 'immunoglobulins' that give us the power to fight against diseases, especially infections from viruses and bacteria (the antigens), as in the case of the common cold, influenza, acute bronchitis etc. When we develop an infection, our immune system gets the message which, in turn, leads to an antibody response. Normally, this will help fight the attack by the

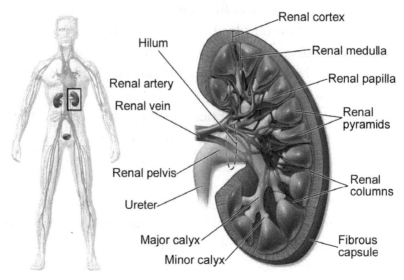

Kidney Anatomy

Figure 1. Normal Kidney Anatomy: Image courtesy of Blausen. wcom staff (2014). "Medical gallery of Blausen Medical 2014." Wikijournal of Medicine 1 (2). DOI:10.15347/wjm/2014.010. ISSN 2002-44

antigens (infection) and restore the body back to health. This is our defense system. The various types of immunoglobulins are commonly designated as IgG, IgA, IgD and IgM. Quantitatively, IgA is the most dominant immunoglobulin produced in the human body.

The basic functional unit in the kidney is called a nephron. Glomerulus, consisting of a capillary tuft, is the main filtering component of the nephron, the site where many of the waste products in the body and excess body water are eliminated as urine. And this is where IgA gets deposited. Although our immune system with its ability to produce an antibody (such as IgA) response to foreign antigens is meant to protect the body from the hostile attack of antigens, sometimes this function goes awry and our own native Ig A attacks our own kidneys and gets deposited in the glomeruli. This is a very puzzling phenomenon that leads to inflammation followed by destruction of the renal tissue! IgA N is considered an autoimmune disease because the primary defect is in the immune system. It leads to blood and protein leaking into the urine (hematuria and albuminuria), high blood pressure, swollen hands and feet, and other signs of chronic kidney disease. Finally, the process results in total renal failure needing renal replacement therapy in the form of dialysis or transplantation.

At first, the disease was believed to be of little threat. But after more and more researchers looked into IgA N, it turned out that as many as 50% of the cases progressed to end stage renal disease (ESRD) resulting in kidney failure. Currently, IgA N is the third leading cause of chronic kidney disease in the United States after diabetes and high blood pressure. In Japan and France, the incidence of the disease is twice as that found in USA; therefore testing for the condition is part of regular preventive medical care. In USA, however, this is rarely performed as a preventive measure. Most people probably never realize they have the disease until late, when renal function has gone down significantly. Amongst those diagnosed as having IgA N, as many as 20% - 30% will suffer eventual kidney failure within 10-20 years and will require life-saving dialysis and/or a kidney transplant."

While doing pediatric rotation during my medical school days, I had seen many cases of nephrotic syndrome. Whenever a child was brought in with a puffy face and swelling of the feet and ankles, we would remark to each other with a touch of sadness, "Oh, here is another case," knowing full well that no specific cure existed for the disease. Diuretics helped to get rid of some fluid. Fortunately, many of them turned out to have self-limiting disease and eventually made a complete recovery but a few succumbed to the disease. A lot of them came from poor families and suffered from streptococcal (bacterial) skin infections, thought to be a common precursor of this disease in those days. We hadn't heard about IgA nephropathy nor did we have the facility to do renal biopsy at that time. Most likely many of these children suffered from IgA N

~~~

All the nephrologists whom I consulted felt that my IgA N may have been progressing for some time without my knowledge. Although the diagnosis was confirmed by a tissue biopsy, I was still somewhat skeptical. So, I had the slides reviewed again by a close friend of mine, Dr. Selvi Gunasekharan, a senior pathologist at Tampa General Hospital.

"Ravi, there is no question about the diagnosis," she said. "In fact, I see the tell-tale changes in a fairly good number of the glomeruli in the slide."

"What does that mean?" I asked anxiously.

"Well, it suggests significant involvement of the kidneys. Definitely not early stage," she said, confirming Dr. Pardo's report. It intrigued me to no end that I could come down with such an exotic disease that primarily affected children. Although I had no reason to disbelieve the verdict of two eminent pathologists that corroborated the clinical manifestations of my disease, I still needed to convince myself in no uncertain terms about the diagnosis. So the slides were sent to NIH (National Institute of Health), the ultimate authority in all medical matters, for final review.

Not surprisingly, the reply from NIH was exactly the same as the previous reports! There was no question about the diagnosis or the extent of its progression. What a miserable let down! "You better accept the diagnosis and move on," I said to myself. Kidneys normally cope with many of the insults thrown at them for a while, but once it reaches the tipping point, they start failing and the serum creatinine starts rising. Persistent elevation of serum creatinine is an automatic indication that the kidney function is reduced to half. This meant that, unbeknownst to me, my disease had been ravaging my poor kidneys for some time.

Suddenly, everything made sense. The little albuminuria noted during routine testing a few years ago was indeed the harbinger of an illness that had become fully manifest now. Dr. DeVelasco and Dr. Mars both informed me that there was no specific treatment for this condition. The only way to slow the progression of the disease would be to control my hypertension and stay on a low-salt, low-protein diet. "The value of a low-protein diet is not established yet. But we could put you on our clinical trials – MDRD study (Modification of Diet in Renal Diseases)," said Dr Mars during my next follow-up in Gainesville. I opted out of the study, not seeing any necessity to be part of a research at this time.

How would you react when you suddenly realize that your life is threatened with an incurable illness? In my mind, there was some mystique to this illness. No one in my family or friendship circle or even among my acquaintances had ever been diagnosed with it. I still struggled with the "Why me?" question at this unexpected illness. At times, I just couldn't curb the onslaught of philosophical thoughts rising in my brain. Finally I reconciled to the fact that *nature* makes unilateral decisions and we simply have to abide by its rules. As one author put it, "There is randomness in everything in the universe. So it can strike you as much as anybody else, any time."

My wife continued to reassure me by instilling confidence to move forward. "Dialysis or transplant, whatever is the right approach, we will handle it when the time comes," she said, trying to hide her own welling tears.

When I checked the hemodialysis registry of USA, only 1.2% of the nearly 122,000 people who were undergoing dialysis were Asians. In fact, I knew no other Indians in my acquaintance who suffered from this disease, nor was anybody on dialysis. Then I remembered reading an article in Reader's Digest that said, "When God gives you a problem, He also gives you the necessary wisdom and tools to solve it." I sincerely hoped that was true, although I couldn't immediately think of any solutions.

The dark vision of impending renal failure gave me insomnia and nightmares, but I tried to avoid sleeping pills, though recommended for temporary use by my physicians to tide over my current mental turmoil. Non-steroidal anti-inflammatory drugs like ibuprofen that can be harmful to the kidneys were carefully avoided. Finally, I decided to get my life back in order and move forward.

Being primarily a vegetarian, sticking to a low-protein diet wasn't difficult. I followed the low-salt-protein-restricted diet to a fault, ordering such food items from out-of-state suppliers, exercised regularly and controlled my hypertension well. The work schedule was reorganized, careful not to overload myself. Traveling ninety miles to Gainesville every three months for follow-up appointments was not easy, especially with a busy practice. So I established as a patient with Dr. Samuel Weinstein in Tampa, a transplant nephrologist, Tampa being closer.

During my first visit, I asked him the same old tiresome question that I had asked all my other doctors before, "How much time do I have before I go into renal failure?"

"Oh, come on, Dr. Nathan, don't worry about those things," Sam reassured me. "You know every patient is different. When that time comes, we will give you a new kidney." He said it with such lightheartedness, as though it was an everyday procedure, in an effort to put me at ease! We shared a laugh.

"A renal transplantation! Well, easier said than done," I mumbled to myself. In fact, I could see that not-so-distant possibility already looming on the horizon.

4

Adapting to New Circumstances

April, 1989

THE NEXT SEVERAL weeks saw me intermittently brooding over my illness while I started to make the necessary mental adjustments in order to do my work as a cardiologist. I felt fine physically and my hypertension was well controlled with small doses of two medicines, lisinopril and metoprolol. Previously, I was only taking one drug, lovastatin, for my high cholesterol. The thought of having to take an assortment of medications starting in the not-too-distant future and perhaps for the rest of my life made me miserable, but now I could empathize with my sick patients on multiple drugs.

The strict diet I had to follow didn't bother me much, but Susheela had to prepare special dishes. I have always advocated a low-salt diet to my patients because of the close association between high salt intake and hypertension. The average American consumes more than 3.5 gm of salt daily although we need only less than 2.0 gms. I was also fascinated with the example of the *Maasai* tribe, an ethnic group of semi-nomadic pastoral people inhabiting Kenya and northern Tanzania, in whom hypertension is virtually non-existent because they do not use any salt at all.

I continued to read as much medical articles on IgA N as I could find. Dr. Mars sent me a chapter from one of the recent text books, and I collected a few other publications. All these said the disease is more common in Europeans, especially within the French and Mediterranean littoral.

"Maybe you are of European descent, who knows?" Susheela joked one day. "We need to check your ancestry. Your hair is a little brownish, and your complexion is fairer than that of an average Indian." As a pediatrician, she knew more about this disease. "But most of these children get better, unlike the adults," she added. Well, that wasn't much comfort.

"Unfortunately, I am not a child anymore," I said wistfully.

"But you certainly act like one sometimes; that may be a blessing in disguise, for a better prognosis perhaps," she commented jokingly to buoy my spirits.

Some of the traits of the disease did bother me. Apparently, if there is gross *hematuria* in the urine (visible blood in the urine), the prognosis is good! Unfortunately, with microscopic hematuria like mine, the prognosis isn't so great. As a rule, in adult patients, when gross hematuria is detected, doctors get very concerned, immediately thinking of something like cancer of the kidney. Whereas, in cases of IgA N, at least one-fourth of patients with microscopic hematuria will end up in renal failure during the next few years! That was a frightening thought.

~~~

My physician friends who specialized in nephrology had to field several calls from me as I desperately tried to understand the disease better. They were, of course, very helpful, saying my disease was more likely to be only slowly progressive, and that I shouldn't worry too much at this stage. But the unanimous opinion was, sooner or later, I would be in renal failure. One gave me just three years before needing dialysis, so I decided it was time to reconcile with my situation. This is beyond my control; I can't act like a patient when I have to continue my career as a doctor.

The entire focus of my life had been my family and the large cardiovascular practice I had built over the past eight years. There was a lot of responsibility on my shoulders since my son, Sandeep (we call him Dipu), had started his seven year BS/MD honors program at Boston University, and Sanu, was still in middle school and had a long way to go. So I had to quickly adapt myself to the new circumstances and move on; whatever was destined to happen will happen and had to be faced courageously.

More than physical symptoms, emotional upheavals still raised their ugly heads occasionally. So I contacted a psychologist who specialized in bio-feedback techniques to decide if my hypertension could be controlled without medications but his techniques failed on me. After the first session, both of us decided there was nothing wrong with my mind. The high blood pressure resulted from an organic disease that would need proper therapy. So I abandoned any more research on mind control and resorted to simple meditation in the morning for a few minutes that gave me some peace of mind. Initial anxieties over, I was now ready to face the illness in the most practical way with the help of my physicians, family and friends.

Periodic clinical check-ups, a quick run to the local lab for blood tests, calling them to get the results the following day and frequent discussions with the nephrologist became part of my daily routine. A rise in the level of creatinine, in my blood is considered the benchmark for progression of kidney disease. Fortunately, after six months, it had remained steady, hovering around 2.2. For now, the current treatment seemed to work.

My professional work kept me very busy and there were a lot of family responsibilities. Initially, I thought of slowing down a bit. But

I changed my mind since I felt up to speed. Sitting at home idly has never been an option for me. I didn't want to allow myself any chance to dwell on future complications. Twelve-hour work days, weekend calls, emergency consults and frequent trips to ICU and CCU, at times in the middle of the night, again became part of my routine. I worked as though I had to prove something to myself and to everyone else! In a true fighting spirit, I wanted to make sure that this "unwelcome intruder" hadn't disabled me, yet hoping to arrest the progression of the disease by some miracle.

Only a few of my close friends knew that I was battling a progressive renal disease. With reinforced resolve, I stuck to my special diet, played tennis twice weekly with my buddy and neighbor, Dr. Paul, and jogged three miles at least twice weekly. I re-read Norman Vincent Peale's 'Power of Positive Thinking.' Luckily, there were no further setbacks and the year went by smoothly, with the creatinine level staying around 2.2 and BP under control. I even started playing some competitive tennis, participating in the 45-plus category, mostly fundraisers for the American Cancer Society and American Heart Association (AHA), reaching the semifinals of the AHA charity tournament once!

"Not bad for a cardiologist suffering from IgA Neprhropathy," complimented my wife who was in the bleachers applauding my shots.

5

A NEW TWIST

February 8, 1990

JUST WHEN I *had settled into a smooth routine envisioning no major problems on the horizon, something new and unpleasant happened.*

One day while playing tennis, I felt a little twinge of pain in my chest. Could this be angina (pain resulting from decreased blood flow to the heart muscle or *coronary artery disease* – CAD). I knew I was at high risk for CAD because of my high cholesterol and hypertension, although both were under good control. There were sporadic reports that an increase in the creatinine levels may be an independent risk factor for CAD, and mine remained stable, albeit elevated, around 2.4 for several months now.

The next day I met with Dr. B.R. Raju, my colleague, the senior cardiologist at our hospital and a good friend; and apprised him of my new complaints. He immediately suggested an exercise stress test with stress echocardiogram. I enumerated my risk factors; my father had a heart attack when he was sixty nine and later died of a stroke at

75. One of my older brothers had developed angina at 58 and now I am beginning to feel angina-like symptom. Is it my turn now? Soon I found myself taking the proverbial exercise stress test, the Bruce Test that I myself have administered to a few thousand patients in the past.

The Bruce Test is a treadmill exercise stress test to evaluate patients with suspected coronary heart disease. Simultaneous EKG tracings are obtained at rest and during and after exercise to see if there are changes suggestive of myocardial ischemia in response to the exercise. Since the predictive accuracy of a treadmill stress test alone is not great, it is often combined with cardiac imaging, either a nuclear scan with radio-isotopes, like Thallium or Sestamibi, or, an echocardiogram that shows ultrasound images of the heart.

The tech said the lab was ready and waiting. I got on the treadmill with all the leads and electrodes connected to different parts of my body and hooked on to the EKG monitor. A blood pressure cuff was fitted around my left arm. I completed ten minutes of exercise using the standard Bruce protocol that took me to 4.0 miles per hour at a 16-degree incline. The last minute was difficult, but I managed to reach a metabolic level of 10, generally acceptable for a 50-year old guy. The echo technician took several images of my heart before, during and after the exercise.

I completed the entire exercise without any angina. The EKG response wasn't quite characteristic of myocardial ischemia (reduced blood flow) but showed some minor non-specific changes in some leads. "Let us review these images," Dr. Raju said looking at the echo monitor screen and running the video loop back and forth. "See this area, Ravi," he said pointing to the apex and adjoining septal region of the heart in the four chamber view. "There is some motion abnormality, the region is almost hypokinetic (weakly contracting), may be even dyskinetic (abnormally contracting), don't you think?" he asked me.

I knew the implications. *Hypokinesia* and *dyskinesia* are wall motion abnormalities observed on the cardiac muscle as it contracts and relaxes. When seen during a stress test, they often represent some kind of blockage in the coronaries. Since I didn't have any persistent symptoms like angina on exertion, shortness of breath or fatigue, and nothing interfered with my general work performance, Dr. Raju felt medical treatment was all I needed for now and I agreed. "Take some beta blockers, baby aspirin and continue with your *lisinopril*; stay on the low-fat diet and your current exercise pattern," he suggested.

"We have to call this a positive stress test and maybe repeat it after six months, assuming you don't have any further symptoms," Dr. Raju cautioned.

"I couldn't have serious coronary disease," I had reassured myself earlier. Well, I was in denial! However, after the test, I decided to stop playing vigorous tennis. Who wants to challenge the ticker? Deep down, I had a feeling that something wasn't quite right with my heart.

6

ESCALATING CARDIAC PROBLEM

Wednesday, June 27, 1990

LITTLE DID I realize this would turn out to be a fateful day in my life. In the morning, I got ready for work but first walked around the driveway and enjoyed some fresh country air saturated with the fragrance of the jasmines, roses and gardenias growing abundantly in our garden. A herd of deer took flight across the back fence, sensing my presence. Feeling good, I drove to the hospital; the first stop would be the ICU.

Halfway through the four-mile drive to the hospital, I felt a little chest discomfort, but discounted angina as a possibility, perhaps in denial. I should have known better, having had a positive stress test only two months ago. Holding the wheel steady, I took my own pulse. It was regular with no extra beats which was slightly reassuring since frequent extra beats or *ventricular ectopics* occur if the heart muscle is suffering from ischemia as happens often during an episode of angina or heart attack.

Since February I had been paying even more attention to my diet and exercise, walking 20–30 minutes almost daily at a steady pace. Of course, I had stopped doing anything too strenuous and took my medications diligently. Yet my intuition told me that I'd better check into the Emergency Room (ER) right away. My wife arrived in a few minutes, unconcealed panic etched on her face.

The next thing I knew, I was lying in a patient bed, wearing a hospital gown, hooked up to an overhead cardiac monitor, two intravenous lines in place, oxygen being given through the nostrils via a nasal cannula and a bunch of nurses and doctors with solemn faces hovering around me. The ER doctor, after a brief evaluation, called Dr. Raju and I was quickly whisked away to the CCU. Although the EKG was inconclusive, Dr. Raju felt I was developing a cardiac event, most likely unstable angina and needed close observation. I realized that I would be going to the CCU as a patient today, not as a cardiologist!

No doubt, the doctor's lounge would be abuzz with the breaking news, *"Did you hear about Dr. Nathan?"* During visiting hours, my twelve-year-old daughter came to see me and declared that this might even lead to *schadenfreude,* which means pleasure in the misfortune of others. She was preparing for her forthcoming spelling bee competition and loved to use a new word whenever possible. I told her, "I don't have any enemies here, if anything, they would be more concerned about themselves, knowing this can happen to them as well."

While spending time as patient #5 in the CCU, watching the green wavy lines of the electrocardiogram through the corners of my eyes, I wondered how many of my colleagues, successful immigrants from India who had entered this land of plenty, might have gone through this same process. Nearly every day I'd heard horror stories of Indian men and a few non–Indian immigrants as well, having a heart attack or coronary bypass surgery, some even dying suddenly in the prime of their lives.

A few recent studies published in respected medical journals had highlighted that the risk for heart attacks (CAD or coronary artery disease) is quite high in Indian male immigrants in the U.S. My good friend, Dr. E. A. Enas, a prominent cardiologist in Chicago, had studied this problem in depth. His *Coronary Artery Study in Indians (CADI)* had received a lot of attention in the medical media, especially among the Indian circles. I also knew that similar studies from Singapore, East London and South Africa had arrived at the same conclusion. All attributed this high risk for CAD in Indians to their special type of cholesterol abnormalities (low levels of HDL or good cholesterol and high levels of LDL or bad cholesterol). These much-publicized facts about premature coronary artery disease among Indians and their frequent deaths after immigration had been a cause for concern.

Biding my time in the ER bed doing nothing, introspection got the better of me. "What am I doing wrong? Look at me, here I am in the hospital grappling with multiple serious health issues," I asked myself. For most of us professionals, life is a continuous cycle of hospital rounds, procedures, lunch-on-the-run, heavy office schedules, committee meetings, CME (Continuing Medical Education) conferences and more, all resulting in a ceaseless adrenaline rush. Throw in your PRO (Peer Review Organization) denials, problems with billing and collection, troublesome office employees, letters from malpractice attorneys, legal depositions and requests for record release from patients – the scenario for high degree of stress is complete. Even letters from the usually polite medical records department periodically take on a vicious look like *"Your hospital privileges will be suspended if you don't complete your charts in twenty four hours!"*

Later in the day, my second EKG and the other test results came back. Fortunately, there was no evidence of an acute heart attack but the typical symptoms, my high-risk status and some EKG changes suggested that I may be having a *pre-infarction angina*, a forerunner of a heart attack. Dr. Raju suggested I undergo a cardiac catheterization (*cath* for short), a special test to evaluate the status of my coronaries and identify blocks, if any. So I was transferred to the Regional Medical Center at Bayonet Point, which was only thirty miles away, that same afternoon. Dr. Raju was gracious enough to ride with me and Susheela in the ambulance to Bayonet Point.

Dr. Rao Musunuru, my good friend and a senior cardiologist at Bayonet Point Heart Institute, examined me as soon as I arrived and scheduled a cardiac catheterization for the following morning. I felt comfortable in the telemetry unit where I was admitted for observation. Having had a stressful day so far, I dozed off, relieved to be in good hands.

7

〰〰〰

Emergency!

Wednesday, June 27, 1990

It was about 5:00 p.m. I was resting comfortably in bed number two under the watchful eyes of the friendly nurses. With all the drugs on board including beta blockers, nitro pills, BP and cholesterol medications, oxygen and more, everything seemed to have stabilized for now. Or so I thought.

Then I began to feel more chest pains. To my horror, I could see some changes in my EKG tracing on the overhead monitor. The ST segment on the monitor lead was beginning to shift upwards. I was sure that wasn't a good sign, it indicated something worse than angina. "Am I developing a heart attack, after all?" I wondered. Instinctively, as a cardiologist, I knew these changes seemed to point toward *Prinzmetal's* angina—a special variety that portends an impending heart attack, a scary diagnosis. It was, indeed, an emergency. One blow after another was raining down on me! I asked Ron, my nurse, to alert Dr. Musunuru right away.

"Don't worry," he said. "I will give you a nitro pill to put underneath your tongue now. That should take care of the pain. You are scheduled for a cardiac cath in the morning." He didn't seem to be too concerned about the pain and left to attend sicker patients. But knowing the gravity of this newest development, I wasn't about to let it go until morning. No time to lose here.

"Oh no, the chest pains are really bad," I asserted politely. "Could you *please* inform my cardiologist right away?" I wanted an emergency cardiac catheterization and intervention, if indicated. Worried to the hilt, Susheela intervened and had Dr. Musunuru paged. Lucky for me, the hardworking, dedicated cardiologist was still making his evening rounds in the hospital. He quickly rushed over to my bedside and concurred with my thoughts. After a few anxious moments, the ball started rolling.

It was almost 8:00 p.m. The whole atmosphere in the telemetry unit had changed drastically. The place was soon abuzz with action. Frantic calls were made to Dr. Musunuru's associate, Dr. Zaki, the interventional cardiologist, the nurse in charge of the cath lab and the cath technician. They needed to come down to the hospital immediately and get the lab ready. Emergency cardiac catheterizations, especially after hours, were rarely undertaken and the floors were not quite geared for such eventualities at that time.

The cardiac surgeon, Dr. Vijay, was called for surgical back up, as part of the protocol for any emergency coronary interventions. In case the angioplasty failed or resulted in complications that would need emergency coronary bypass surgery, the cardiac surgical team should be ready. He called back promptly and said, "No problem. I'll come any time you want me there." He and I had been longtime friends.

One of the techs came to get my consent for the procedure. Dr. Reddy was informed and he ordered the nurse to give me intravenous *mucomyst (N-acetylcysteine)* to protect my kidneys before the iodinated contrast material used for coronary angiogram was injected. Meanwhile, my pain had escalated and I sweated profusely; so I received a couple of doses of morphine.

By 10:00 p.m., I was wheeled into the cardiac cath suite where the nurse and tech were all set to go. Many of my friends had assembled in the waiting area. Susheela was trembling like a leaf, terrified and feeling helpless, being fully cognizant of the looming contingency. A strange calm had descended on me, and I uttered a few prayers. Dr. Zaki, I knew, was one of the best in the business. Within a few minutes, I was gently helped onto the cath table, my groin cleaned and prepped with *betadine*. The small amount of IV *Versed* given for sedation helped me, but I did not fall asleep. I could feel the skin being injected with a local anesthetic. From then on, it was smooth sailing.

I craned my neck to see the fluoroscopic images as they started appearing on the screen. Dr. Zaki inserted the coronary catheter through the special sheath into the artery in the right leg and snaked it up the abdominal aorta, gently guiding it into the mouth of the left main coronary artery and injected some dye. I could sense the muffled excitement in the room as they watched the dye coursing through the two branches—the large artery in the front wall of the heart called left anterior descending (LAD) and the one that goes around the heart, the circumflex artery. (Coronary arteries supply blood to the heart muscle and consist of a left main segment that divides into LAD and circumflex arteries; they are the source of blood supply to two-thirds of the heart muscle. The right coronary or RCA has a separate origin from the right side of aortic root – see Figure 3) He injected the dye a couple of times into the LAD and then reviewed the instant display on the screen.

"Ravi, you have a tight lesion in the proximal LAD," he said in typical cardiologist's lingo as he pointed to the near total occlusion in the artery on the video (Figure 2). "There may be a clot there as well. We need to either do a quick angioplasty or give tPA," he added.

What this meant in layman's terms is that I had a serious block in the artery that supplies blood to the entire front wall of the heart (Figure 1). "tPA" or *tissue plasminogen activator*, a clot buster, could be used to open up the artery but it can cause serious bleeding, sometimes in the brain, causing strokes. Angioplasty, also called PTCA (Percutaneous Transluminal Coronary Angioplasty) for short, involves dilating the coronary artery with a balloon-tipped catheter inserted via the femoral vein. Although done mostly as an elective procedure, it was gaining acceptance as an emergency procedure for the treatment of acute heart attacks and impending heart attacks. Bayonet Point Hospital had only just started doing this procedure at that time.

Dr. Zaki was very concerned about me; an instantaneous decision had to be made. He debated which one of the alternatives would be most beneficial. We already knew tPA was effective, at best only in 70 to 80% cases whereas an emergency PTCA was superior to prevent an impending heart attack. A heart attack from a block in the LAD will result in considerable damage to the heart, often resulting in death. Hence the LAD artery was often referred to as the "widow maker." So, I told him to go right ahead with angioplasty. Even in my foggy state, I was aware of the seriousness of my problem and my anxiety rose to galactic levels.

For the next several minutes, my life hung in the balance. The special balloon catheter was advanced to an area beyond the lesion in the LAD and the balloon was inflated. Instantaneously, I felt the unmistakable chest pain of angina, from a temporary cessation of the blood flow through the area. Dr. Zaki quickly deflated and withdrew the catheter, and I received some morphine for relief of pain. He did two more dilatations and was satisfied with the outcome.

"Looks good, Ravi," he said happily. I could sense his smile beneath the mask, satisfied with the results of his efforts.

"Thank God! I don't have any chest pains now," I said in a groggy, muffled voice.

He pulled out the catheter from the groin, but kept the sheath in the artery as a precautionary measure, in case he had to go back and do the procedure again since the dilated area of the artery can close up occasionally, necessitating an emergency angioplasty. The sheath was pulled out later in the ICU when everything appeared to be stable and pressure applied for a few minutes. Now I could breathe easy, I told myself. I mentally thanked Dr. Andreas Gruentzig, the Swiss cardiologist who first developed this technique of balloon angioplasty in Zurich that had saved thousands of lives already.

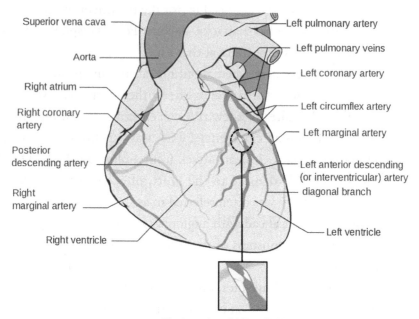

Blockage in middle of LAD artery

Illustration adapted from Patrick J. Lynch, Wikimedia Commons

Figure 2: Coronary Artery Disease: Occlusion in the Left Anterior Descending Artery (like the one I had)

The rest of the day was uneventful and I kept my light dinner down without nausea or vomiting. However, around 3:00 a.m., I woke up and found myself lying in a pool of blood. The site in my right thigh where they punctured the artery for catheterization was bleeding profusely, and I had lost some blood. The bed sheets were soaked. The nurses were supposed to check my wound periodically and observe for complications. I buzzed my nurse urgently. Fortunately, the bleeding was controlled promptly and no transfusion was needed.

Everyone, including Dr. Zaki and I, was worried about my kidney function since so much dye had been injected. In my dazed state, I had some difficulty passing urine, so they inserted a Foley catheter into my bladder. I had no idea that this would later result in some of the worst moments of my life from a severe urinary infection.

The following morning, I felt better and later in the day I went with Dr. Zaki to see the coronary angiograms myself and only then realized the gravity of the crisis. I was so close to suffering a severe heart attack! The LAD had a 99% block and it was only minutes before a catastrophe could have occurred. Then I came back to my bed and quickly dozed off.

"Open your eyes, see who's here!" I heard the nurse saying cheerfully. There he was, like an angel—Dipu, our son. He had taken the first flight he could get. What a relief!

I went home on the third day, quite happy about the outcome, but soon developed a severe, painful urinary infection, no doubt induced by the Foley catheter. The agony and discomfort were unbearable during the next several days, worse than all my previous ailments. Finally, with a lot of antibiotics, oral fluids and rest, everything improved and I was back to my normal self again.

Typically, we worry about developing one serious disease, something that can threaten our life. But how do you manage two severe diseases – IgA N and serious heart disease simultaneously? That was my predicament after going through the ordeals of the past few months. I knew I had to implement a lot more discipline and control in my life to prevent the progression of both diseases, my biggest challenge yet. This meant even a stricter diet, regular exercise, more cholesterol-reducing drugs and a stress-free life too. The last one, while in cardiology practice, would be a pipe dream; but realizing that I had been given a reprieve this time, I vowed to try harder with reinforced resolve.

8

———— ∿∿ ————

What Next?

August, 1990

Ever since the diagnosis of IgA N the only thought in my mind was how best to slow down the progression of this disease. Apparently, there were multiple mechanisms by which the innocent kidney becomes a silent victim to the attack of this deadly immune complex. Recurrent virus infections or allergies have been cited as a cause of stimulation of the immune system in many patients.

Two factors exacerbated my anxiety. Once considered benign, IgA N is not; many with only low grade urinary abnormalities at the onset, would inexorably progress to severe renal insufficiency. Secondly, IgA N is among the most common causes of end-stage renal failure. I was a little dejected as it seemed there was no way to escape my fate.

Looking back, I could remember getting frequent upper respiratory infections during my cardiology fellowship days at the New Jersey College of Medicine. Working in the cardiac catheterization lab as well as the experimental dog lab, I was exposed to a significant degree of radiation. The research project assigned to me by Dr. Tim Regan, the Director of Cardiology, was to create experimental myocardial infarction (heart attack) in dogs. And this turned out to be a difficult, time-consuming project since I had to negotiate a small catheter into the tiny coronary artery of a beagle under fluoroscopy. The radiation that scattered from the small tower of the X-Ray machine used in the animal lab may have been more than the intended amount.

At one time, my radiation count had exceeded the prescribed limit, and I was taken off the cardiac cath assignment. The Director of Infectious Disease department, Dr Donald Louria whom I consulted, decided after extensive testing that I had come down with a *Coxsackie virus* infection. Although this apparently resolved later, I continued getting frequent bronchitis and wheezing in the winter that necessitated my moving to Florida, which dramatically cured me of those, only to have my allergies flare up, necessitating allergy tests and desensitization shots for five years. Whether all these played a role in the development of my IgA N is anybody's guess.

Thanks to all the research on the disease, one thing became clear. The power of these immune reactants to produce diverse glomerular injury could not be underestimated. And once the injury to the kidney is established, it invariably leads to further inflammatory cellular reactions in the glomeruli, leading to more damage. Proteins, mainly albumin, and blood seep into the little renal tubules and get excreted in the urine leading to low levels of serum albumin, hypertension and fluid retention in the body.

I kept telling myself there had to be a cure somewhere hidden in the copies of those numerous publications that had accumulated on my desk. On digging deeper into these research papers and talking to various nephrologists, I was surprised to learn that the relentlessly progressive IgA N, one of the most common forms of kidney diseases in the world, has no known cure as yet! Renal failure (ESRD) is the final endpoint, requiring dialysis or transplantation. Prednisone might be of some value to arrest the disease if it has rapidly progressed. But Dr. Mars didn't think that would be of much benefit in my case. Other solutions of unproven value such as fish oil that contains omega-3 fatty acids was promoted under the rationale that these are known to inhibit the production of certain chemicals like cytokines which might cause glomerular injury. However, the data to support their efficacy has been mixed, at best. Nevertheless, I began taking fish oil capsules for a while, but abandoned it later. Swallowing nearly fifteen capsules a day wasn't exactly thrilling. I wondered if I started smelling like a fish!

My next attempt was to try to get a feel of what would be my clinical course and prognosis for the future. Judging from the vast amount of literature I read, the clinical course could fall anywhere on a spectrum between rapid deterioration to renal failure, or slow progression over the next eight to ten years. Opinions were mixed among my many nephrology friends. The more I read, the more I realized, there was no typical clinical course for this disease.

After three consultations from three different university groups, I finally reconciled to the idea that there is no evidence-based curative treatment for this condition. So all I could hope was to preserve the current level of kidney function for some more time with good control of hypertension and healthy lifestyle. I didn't want to give in to the pessimistic thoughts about an uncertain future. I would grab the bull by its horns when it showed up.

I learned how to manipulate my dietary protein as part of the conservative management of renal disease by getting rid of animal protein as much as possible and reducing the protein load. Red meat became a taboo in our house. Shortly after starting all these dietary adjustments, the nationwide MDRD trial was completed and the surprising conclusion was "Reducing protein intake did not significantly delay the rate of decline in kidney function in patients with renal insufficiency!" However, many nephrologists and some research papers attested to the opposite view, so I decided that the best option for me was to go on a moderate protein diet along with the other measures like controlling my BP etc. already implemented.

9

SUDDENLY, A NEW COMPLICATION!

September 25, 1990

FOR A WHILE, I felt well. At least the initial concerns of the new disease had abated. Yet every time my blood tests were due, I would experience moments of anxiety, wondering if my creatinine had gone up. Fortunately it stabilized around 3 mg/dl, only a bit higher than before.

Although the BP was under control, my potassium levels often ran afoul. It hit a critical level of 7 mg/dl one day, nearly double the normal value – a condition called *hyperkalemia*. This is very dangerous to the heart since it can induce serious rhythm disorders including sudden cardiac arrest! And to think I was playing vigorous tennis the previous day with this degree of hyperkalemia made me shudder with fright because strenuous exercise can release more potassium from the muscles into the blood, elevating it to risky levels. Maybe that was what happened.

"Talk about living dangerously!" said Susheela who was very worried about this new development. "You should avoid your favorite bananas and oranges now, they are loaded with potassium." Anyway, after I changed lisinopril (known to increase potassium levels in the blood) to a different one, *amlodipine (Norvasc)*, a calcium channel blocker, the potassium level came down to a comfortable level. That was a big relief.

My stamina was still quite good. I started playing tennis regularly and jogging a couple of miles twice a week again. Believe it or not, I even won my first tournament in the local 50-plus category, organized for the benefit of the American Heart Association. I was already back to my full work schedule. My mental anguish had vanished considerably, and I didn't get upset with the little nuisances in life anymore.

One day, I suddenly felt a little pain in my left shoulder which took me by surprise.

"Could this be tendinitis associated with your tennis?" asked my wife.

"But I play tennis with my right hand. If anything, the right shoulder should be the sore one," I argued.

"Could this be gout?" I wondered. I knew my uric acid levels in the blood had been high, often around 9-10 mg/dl (normal being 3-7 mg/dl), a condition called *hyperuricemia,* the main culprit in the production of *gout (podagra).* But the shoulder is the least commonly affected joint. Gout seems to pick the joints in the feet, especially the big toes, ankles, knees and hands more often.

"It's rare to see gout in renal failure, in spite of high uric acid," my nephrologists opined. So I decided not to worry about it. I was already on a low protein diet, which is good for gout. The pains subsided after a couple of days and I forgot about the incident altogether.

A few days later, I woke up in the middle of the night with intense pain and tenderness in my right big toe. The agonizing pain increased by the minute and pretty soon, my toe was on fire! Everything fit the classic text book description of gout—"Satan's wand touching your big toe which immediately becomes red hot, swollen, exquisitely painful and sensitive, even to rubbing against the bed sheet." I screamed in pain. I took some *Tylenol* first, later aspirin and *Darvocet* too, with hardly any relief. Finally, I called the nephrologist on call who conceded this had to be gout and suggested that I take *Indocin*, a non-steroidal anti-inflammatory drug that would give some relief, but could damage the kidney further. "The harmful effect is usually reversible if you take it for only two or three days," my doctor assured me. So, I tried *Indocin,* and in a few hours the pain improved. I had to hop around the hospital during rounds and pretend that I aggravated an old tennis injury since I didn't want anybody to know that I was disabled with gout. The nurses bought that explanation. Later, I was started on a drug called *Zloprim* (allopurinol) to bring down the high uric acid levels in the blood. I continued to improve and the serum uric acid steadily came down. This was another unwelcome visitor into my ailing body.

All was quiet for the next two months. I even considered stopping the allopurinol for a while. My nephrologists were still puzzled about my gout attacks since I didn't fit the typical mold for gout; I was of thin build, loyal to a near-vegetarian diet and had no family history of gout. Nor was I taking any medicines that would trigger gout. My alcohol consumption was limited to an occasional glass of wine during a party. Maybe it was all related to my kidney disease.

But the next attack, I will remember as long as I live.

Early one morning, I woke up from a deep sleep with intense pain, swelling, tenderness and warmth in the right knee joint. It was literally on fire, I really thought Satan was standing next to my bed, touching my knee with his vicious blazing wand.

"Oh my God!" I let out an ear-piercing cry. For a moment, I didn't realize what had hit me. Maybe I was bitten by a scorpion or a centipede, not uncommon in Florida.

"What is it now? Why all this racket?" my wife complained. "It is way past midnight, you know,"

"It's my knee, my knee…it's on fire!" I wailed. "Boy, this is a vicious pain, terribly tender too! Believe me, it's unbearable."

"Switch on the reading lamp. Let me look at it," she said. The illuminated digital clock said it was 3:00 a.m.

As soon as the light came on, I could see my right knee was very swollen, warm and tender to the touch – classic signs of acute arthritis that could only mean gout. In spite of taking preventive measures including allopurinol, and even with the serum uric acid being normal, my gout had returned. Now I had no option other than going to the hospital ER to get an injection for fast relief.

The ER doctor promptly gave me an injection of *colchicine*, both as a diagnostic and a therapeutic measure. He drew my blood for complete blood count and uric acid levels. My white cell count was still normal implying no infection which meant this was not septic arthritis. Even the uric acid level was only mildly elevated, not the high levels one might expect after such a fierce attack of gout.

Fortunately, within a few hours after colchicine injection, the pain abated considerably, indirect proof that gout was the diagnosis. The doctor did not suggest a needle aspiration of the knee under local anesthesia to get a sample of the synovial fluid that could have clinched the diagnosis since microscopic examination of the fluid would show the characteristic needle-shaped 'urate crystals,' the diagnostic criterion for gout. But I didn't insist on it either. Later I realized that was a mistake, because a chance for making a definite diagnosis was lost.

"The whole scenario looks like gout. I see this at times with relatively normal uric acid levels, but even that level may be higher for a given person," said Dr. Mohammed Mughni, a reputed rheumatologist in town whom I consulted. Slowly, the diagnosis sank in, and I had to accept the cold facts – one more cross to bear!

I was asked to continue allopurinol and didn't have any further episodes. But it was clear that my whole body was changing, for the worse.

10

10

FAILING KIDNEYS,
MORE PROBLEMS

March, 1994

FIVE YEARS HAD gone by after the diagnosis of my IgA N and I'd been cruising well without any major setbacks. I continued to hope, perhaps foolishly, that the disease had stabilized and wouldn't progress into ESRD (End Stage Renal Disease) and renal failure anytime soon. Unfortunately, hope was about to disappear.

About this time, I developed a little anemia, a decline in my red blood cells (RBCs). This meant that my kidney function was heading further down. This happens because, as the kidney insufficiency progresses, evidenced by a steady increase in the serum creatininine, the level of *erythropoietin,* a hormone produced by the kidney that stimulates the bone marrow to produce red blood cells (RBCs) will gradually go down. RBCs carry the red pigment, hemoglobin (Hb) that transports oxygen to all tissues. Without enough RBCs in the blood, the hemoglobin drops, leading to anemia and resulting in the dysfunction of many organs, including the heart. This shows how many organs are tied to each other in the body.

So I had to start on twice weekly injections of erythropoietin, a brand called *Epogen*. This was a new twist, although I knew most of my patients with significant renal disease were on weekly or biweekly erythropoietin injections. The next six months went by without further developments, and once again, I felt comfortable being the ringmaster of my life.

After the next routine blood tests were done, I got a call from the lab. My creatinine had jumped from 3.2 to a whopping 4.5 in a matter of six months, and the potassium level was also dangerously high—6.9, again! I have seen many patients, with and without renal disease, being brought to the ER with very slow heart rate and low blood pressure, because of hyperkalemia.

Although I didn't feel any different, it was clear that my kidney function was now deteriorating. Inability to maintain normal levels of serum potassium is a red flag and usually means severe kidney dysfunction. After talking this over with Dr. Reddy, I went on a strict low potassium diet and the level, which was monitored often, came down slowly. I secretly hoped that the sudden rise in creatinine could be from a transient setback like an infection or drug effects, and might revert back to the previous levels soon—wishful thinking of a desperate patient again! I was constantly amazed at how my mind, despite being a trained doctor, created these false hopes like so many patients of mine.

"We do see these fluctuations occasionally, but one has to wait and watch," Dr. Reddy cautioned me during my next follow-up visit. "This is also the natural history of the disease, unfortunately," he added. "Once you start losing nephrons for any reason, even if the original disease is under control, the rest of the kidney can't function properly and will continue to deteriorate." He gave me the rationale, "This is unlike many other organs in the body where the remaining healthy tissue can often compensate for the existing damage."

In fact, I was well aware that the natural history of the disease is quite variable and everyone is different in how they respond to the initial treatment. Progression seems to depend more on the severity of the damage in the kidney biopsy but over time most adult patients would get worse and eventually develop kidney failure. Mine had already shown significant kidney damage at the time of initial diagnosis, so this had to be anticipated.

My worst fears were coming true, my dreams of prolonging the kidney function for a while wouldn't be realized. Five years had gone by but it wasn't enough for me. All I could do at this point was to continue the strict regimen and hope the next creatinine level would be better. However, that didn't happen, it steadily climbed to a new peak at 4.9 after a month! At first, I was startled on seeing the report, but I knew it had to be real, since the creatinine clearance (an estimate of kidney function—the lower it is the worse the kidney function is) was also coming down steadily, from around 51 cc/minute five years ago to almost 19.

I didn't know if it was time to inform my relatives in India about my current state of health and not-so-great outlook from here on— whether to press the panic button or not. Even if I downplayed the seriousness of the situation, they would be bewildered. I had a close-knit family and most of the members were very affectionate to each other. But I had a premonition that I was about to face an impending storm. Well, the game was up, I told myself. But the next creatinine level was interestingly down to 4.6! Maybe my IgA N was improving, against all odds, I fantasized.

"Oh, these could be just normal variations," Dr. Reddy said again, putting an end to my line of thinking. "The fact is that your kidney function is showing the expected progression downwards. For now, we will simply watch the lab values and control the blood pressure. Of course, maintain your healthy lifestyle and let us see what happens." What an emotional rollercoaster!

Dr. Reddy was always precise in his views and expressed them gently, so as not to cause any alarm. But he never fudged his answers just to make his patient feel better, either. I always admired him, not only for his profound knowledge in the field, but also for his smooth handling of difficult problems and usually succinct answers to the questions.

My final hope of warding off the onset of the dreadful ESRD for a while shattered with the next blood test a month later - the creatinine had gone up to 5.2! And in another couple of months, it was up to 5.9. I repeated the creatinine clearance and it was down to 13. This meant I would be needing dialysis soon.

"*This is as far as we can take you*," my tired, ailing kidneys seemed to be telling me.

Dr. Ramachandran who arranged my original kidney biopsy in Miami, often gave me second opinions and advice. Whenever I was concerned with an issue, I would call him to get his viewpoint. With the rapidly rising creatinine levels and impending renal failure, Dr. Ramachandran was brought up-to-date regarding my current renal status.

"Do you have any nausea?" he asked.

"Not yet," I said. "My appetite is good, I haven't lost any weight and I can still do my regular exercises."

"Well, that's good. However, your numbers suggest you *are* in End Stage Renal Diseae (ESRD). Many at this stage have some symptoms from the disease and if you do, take soda bicarb." Sodium bicarbonate, an alkali, would counter the metabolic acidosis of ESRD (as the damaged kidneys cannot remove the excess acid from the body and blood becomes more acidotic with a lower pH). He was obviously concerned I might develop *uremic syndrome*, the anticipated complication of ESRD that will need urgent dialysis.

All my physician friends agreed that for my small frame, my actual corrected creatinine may be even higher, which meant *dialysis,* either *hemodialysis or peritoneal dialysis,* was just around the corner! Although I did have some itching of the skin especially in the legs, I didn't quite have any other symptoms of uremia like nausea, vomiting, fatigue etc. So it was decided not to modify the current therapy by including oral intake of any alkali.

11

GETTING READY FOR DIALYSIS

AT THE PRESENT time, the three main life-extending medical treatments available for renal failure patients are "Hemodialysis, Peritoneal dialysis and Renal Transplantation.

Both types of dialysis facilitate the removal of excess fluid and waste products from the body that is characteristic of the disease. In Hemodialysis, a catheter is placed in an arteriovenous fistula (also called A-V shunt), specially fashioned by connecting an artery and the adjoining vein in the arm to make the blood vessels more prominent and accessible to facilitate introduction of dialysis catheters. In Peritoneal Dialysis, the special dialysis fluid (cleansing fluid) flows through a catheter into the abdominal cavity (the lining inside the abdominal cavity called 'peritoneum' acts as a filter) and after a few hours, is drained out; the fluid that comes out would have soaked up all the waste products and excess fluid from the body. This can be done 3-5 times/ day, usually at night during sleep.

Renal transplantation involves getting a new matching kidney – cadaveric or live. There is always a big waiting list for cadaveric donor organs.

Also transplant recipients are vulnerable to complications like rejection, infections, blood clots etc.

Even the very thought of hemodialysis made me nervous although I knew full well it's a life saving treatment for kidney failure. But I wasn't ready to handle the many daily problems a dialysis patient has to face—like frequent hospitalizations, periodic modifications of the A-V shunt (all called A-V fistula, surgical connection between a vein and artery to make the vein bigger, so it can be accessed easily for dialysis), recurrent infections and above all, the disability and fatigue that follows each dialysis session. Having witnessed the misery of many of them, with their days wound around dialysis sessions, I couldn't, for the life of me, imagine being hooked on to a machine three times a week for sessions lasting four to five hours. The procedure is somewhat better now than when dialysis originally started several decades ago and can also be done at home.

Peritoneal Dialysis (PD), the other choice, is a lot simpler, doesn't need any fancy machines and is usually done at home. Many nephrologists consider PD the best initial therapy and this type of homestyle self-care dialysis is better as a long-term therapy as well.

Longevity of both types of dialysis patients is generally shorter than those who receive kidney transplants, the average duration of survival being 9–12 years, depending on several variables. One of our local physicians who was on hemodialysis continued to lead a productive life while practicing for nearly seventeen years before receiving a transplant! But not everyone is that lucky. Blood pressure fluctuations and dizziness from rapid fluid shifts in the body frequently accompany the procedure, requiring emergency hospitalizations. Often patients are so weak, they are at risk for falls, resulting in more problems. The shunt inserted in the forearms for venous access for dialysis can clot, necessitating more surgery that might include repairing or even inserting a new shunt or at the very least, injecting clot-dissolving agents. One of my patients reminded me when I started taking his pulse in the wrist,

"Doc, I am into my third shunt now, so please be careful with my hand."

Some of the recent statistics about ESRD and dialysis also disturbed me very much. According to Dr. Gary E. Striker, a Professor and NIH-funded researcher in kidney diseases and aging, the annual mortality of patients with renal failure persists at more than 20% even with the availability of hemodialysis, primarily because of hypertension, malnutrition and pre⊠dialysis comorbidity. There was also some question whether longer duration of hemodialysis and more frequent dialysis may be associated with better prognosis but apparently there was no consensus among the specialists. What bothered me even more was that the NIDDK (National Institute of Diabetes and Digestive and Kidney Diseases) also cited data indicating the number of ESRD patients was steadily increasing every year. "Maybe transplantation is the best answer," I mused.

One thing was obvious, my life was going downhill. I thought I might go crazy thinking about all the eventualities and was indecisive, now that the time for a major decision had arrived. I felt like I was going down a steep water slide with nothing to hold on to, a fast plunge right ahead for sure. A pall of fear and frustration enveloped me. Being *more* informed about the complications of the disease and its prognosis than my lay counterpart could perhaps generate an even more extreme level of anxiety and tension.

Later in the week, I had an appointment with Dr. Weinstein, and we went over my options in detail. I was careful not to appear overwhelmed by my own emotions. He gave me some pamphlets to read. Basically, I had three options.

1. **Hemodialysis**: This meant a fistula in my arm and going to the dialysis center three times a week. He took a quick look at my left arm to see the status of my veins.
2. **Peritoneal dialysis**. I'd be literally confined to the house for the best part of the day. So, even short weekend travels

would be difficult, carrying all that bulky equipment.

3. *Primary transplantation*: A matching donor has to be found. A living relative would be the best option, followed by living non-related donor and finally, a cadaveric organ. Of course, I would be put on the waiting list for cadaveric transplantation. But with the current problems of organ shortage and long waiting list, my own ethnicity and blood type being O, I could be in for a long wait, at least two years if not more.

"If I had kidney failure, I would opt for peritoneal rather than hemodialysis," Sandy Wilson, the dialysis nurse at my hospital, told me one day. Sandy was a vibrant lady, quite knowledgeable about her patients and cognizant of their feelings. Of course, she didn't know that I was suffering from ESRD and had an ulterior motive in asking many questions. "Hemodialysis isn't so great....they often feel so crummy," she added.

But unbidden images of a peritoneal catheter sticking out of my belly again filled me with horror. What about peritonitis, inflammation of the lining of inner abdomen, which some patients are likely to develop intermittently? After the insertion of peritoneal catheter, I would be forbidden from swimming, an exercise I loved dearly. I may not be allowed to do vigorous exercises like playing tennis, either. Somehow, this option didn't appeal to me very much, even if it was considered to be the better choice. In a pool of indecision, my ambient anxiety raised its frightening head again.

"The best thing for you is a primary transplant," Dr. Reddy said. "You are young, active and the *real treatment for kidney failure is transplantation*. Get your sister here as soon as possible." I realized I could avoid a lot of problems with a transplant.

"Just take three months off, and you can return to work afterwards," he added. "Transplants are simple these days." He was trying to instill some confidence in me.

Surgery? The very thought of somebody cutting my belly open

gave me a shudder and I broke out in a sweat.

"Oh, come on, this is not open heart surgery," Susheela said one day when we were having our umpteenth discussion on the subject. "Where's your grit? Try to be a little brave. So many patients go through this every day all over the world. Didn't you read the pamphlet? This surgery is no more complicated than an inguinal hernia repair. Actually, the donor, your sister, has the major surgery, since the entire kidney has to be removed. Think about her for a moment," she chided me. I felt a little silly and realized that I had no choice in the matter. I certainly didn't want to be hooked to a machine for the rest of my life nor did I want anybody to put catheters into my belly.

"Transplant is the way to go" became my new mantra and I repeated it every day. I was fortunate to have two prospective donors, my two beloved sisters. Yet putting either one of them through the risk of a major surgery made me feel guilty. How could I ask them to donate one of their precious kidneys? But I knew that both of them loved me and wouldn't hesitate even for a moment to give me one of their organs; they had indicated this during my last visit to India, when the subject of my illness came up for discussion and became the main family concern. Even my older brother who was sixty-two had offered to donate one of his kidneys. I felt truly blessed to have a loving and supportive family.

For a brief moment, I marveled at nature's design to give us two kidneys. How lucky we are to have two kidneys? We only need one kidney to live normally. As kidney failure is common in life, the expendability of one kidney makes 'live donor kidney transplantation' a viable option.

12

Journey of a Kidney Donor

June, 1994

Now the most urgent item on my to-do-list was to ask one or both my sisters, the prospective donors, to come to the U.S. For reasons unclear to me, I'd heard the U.S. Consulate in Chennai was sometimes sluggish when giving visas to the U.S. for a prospective traveler; but I thought this would be an easy matter with a certificate from my two nephrologists attesting to the necessity for a live-related donor transplant. It certainly was a life and death issue. My wife and children had a different blood group, A. So I called my older brother Rajappan in India. Though willing to be a donor, his blood group turned out to be B and therefore not a match. He gladly agreed to be the coordinator and do all that is needed at the home front to identify which sister was best suited to be the donor - Ratnam or Thankamani, both of them being of 'O' group, same as mine, and get them a United States visa.

When I gave Ratnam a quick review of my current status and

announced the time for transplant is almost here, she was on the verge of tears.

"Ravi, I didn't know it was this bad. This is a major surgery, right?" she asked.

"Yes *Kochoppol*, it is," I said. "The choice is between dialysis and transplant. Of course, transplant is much better in the long run. But that means I need a donor with a matching blood group."

"I see…" her voice trailed off. She instinctively knew what I meant. It was crunch time now, time for the ultimate sacrifice from one of my sisters. So I told her to inform Thankamani too.

As expected, this triggered a panic reaction among my relatives. Everybody was asking each other, "What's happening to poor Ravi? We thought his illness was under control." To complicate matters, there was a recent death in the family—one of my younger cousins died in a motor vehicle accident. This wasn't a good omen, especially to us, Indians. Of course, nobody wanted to make any negative comment on the eve of my forthcoming surgery. Ratnam was visibly perturbed about my health crisis, but not because she may be called upon to donate one of her kidneys soon. She was full of affection for me and, once said privately,

"Even if something happens to me, it will not be a terrible loss to the family. You are more valuable… you need to live. You are always very productive and you have helped every single member in our family."

"Don't say such things, *Kochoppol*; you are as important as anybody else," I said. "Luckily, removing a kidney from the donor, although a major surgery, is not that complicated. It is easier than removing a slice of the liver (partial hepatectomy) as in liver transplantation."

Ratnam informed all other members right away, "The time for Ravi's transplant surgery is here. No time to lose now. We need to pursue the visa matters urgently as it may take some time."

~~~

In the meantime, my creatinine rose to 6.4. Dr. Reddy asked me to see a vascular surgeon for establishing an AV shunt as a precautionary measure. I had almost daily conversations with Rajappan and he said he would soon be taking both our sisters to the American Consulate in Chennai (Madras). New updated affidavits and supporting certificates were sent to the American Consulate in Chennai to get the ball rolling.

The atmosphere in Thankamani's house on the eve of her travel to Chennai from her home in Changanacherry, Kerala, a mere 400-mile train journey, was a bit tense. Thankamani, a prominent citizen of her town and a senior professor at a major college, had a wide circle of friends. They just couldn't bear the thought of their dear *'Mani'* possibly losing one of her precious organs. Many had assembled there to give her a tearful 'send off.' A few were even skeptical about removal of one of her vital organs and wondered, "Don't know what will happen to her. Will she be disabled for the rest of her life?" I couldn't blame them since transplantation in the early 90s in India was still a novelty and even removal of cadaveric organs was a taboo. So, I could understand the general mindset among relatives and friends there. However, some of them, more knowledgeable about the surgery and its purpose, gave her the much needed moral boost of confidence since she was going to save a life, a very noble gesture indeed!

⤳

My two sisters reported to the American Consulate promptly at 8:00 a.m. and signed their names in the register. As in many other offices, a "first-come, first-served" policy was in force. Although first ones to arrive, the officials kept them waiting until the end of the day and eventually refused the visa for no specific reason. In fact, they didn't even get a chance to see the American Consul. Instead, a rude junior Indian female official came in the afternoon, called Thankamani first, and pelted her with a barrage of questions:

"What is the guarantee your kidney will be matching?" she asked.

"We are of the same blood group, and I am his sister. That's all they want to know," she said confidently.

She tried another technique. "Do you know you can have major complications from this surgery?"

"Excuse me, madam, that is the least of my worries…this is for my dear brother. And it is done in one of the best hospitals in America," she said.

The lady didn't appear to be happy with the answer. She went inside and promptly returned. Clearly, she didn't have the time to consult with the Consul or any senior official, so it was her own decision.

"Your visa is denied. You may go back," she said without any emotion. No explanation, no reasons given, just a blunt statement. Although Thankamani pleaded with the consulate officials several times citing all the reasons for giving her a visa, it was of no avail; they wouldn't budge an inch.

Now it was Ratnam's turn. The official raised the same silly excuses and refused her visa as well. Another reason they cited was, she had overstayed her last visit to the U.S. Instead of six months as originally planned, she did stay for one year, but only after *legally* extending her visitor's visa. No matter how much my sisters pleaded, the consulate staff didn't budge. And both my sisters had foolishly expected congratulations for their willingness to be organ donors!

So after a full day's toil in the consulate, both returned home totally disheartened. All the other applicants that day, including students going for higher studies, some not-so-renowned artists, and many tourists had no problem getting visas! I couldn't believe they would refuse visas to my sisters when they were coming here to save a life—to give a matching kidney to their brother in dire need. So, round one of the visa procurement ended in total failure. This was, indeed, an unexpected turn-around.

Here in Brooksville, I was growing more anxious by the minute, not knowing when my native kidneys would give up completely. If that did happen, acute renal failure will set in and I would need emergency dialysis, something to be avoided.

Ratnam was literally crying when she called me from a pay phone in Madras. "Can you imagine refusing visas to both of us? And they didn't even give us a good reason. I'm so sorry, Ravi," she said. My worst fears had come true, I didn't have a donor! My creatinine was climbing and both Drs. Reddy and Weinstein had asked me to get ready with the arrangements for primary transplant. How was I going to have a transplant if my donor was still in India?

Later in the day, Rajappan took Thankamani to the Apollo Hospital, Chennai, one of the best multispecialty hospitals in India, for a check-up, because of her own concerns regarding her state of health and suitability for the kidney donor surgery. So she used this opportunity to have a full physical and lab work. The nephrologist at Apollo said that her BP was high enough to warrant treatment! She was a bit puzzled since it had always been normal in the past. But repeat measurements confirmed the same finding. Perhaps stress had something to do with it, I felt. The kidney function tests were normal, but she had to take medications to control her new onset hypertension – another twist in the ever-changing saga of my illness that cast doubt on her eligibility to be a donor. However, Ratnam came through all her tests with flying colors and later she would tell me, "Ravi, I was sure I would be found a suitable match; I had sincerely prayed to God for that. That's how much I wanted to donate my kidney to you."

So, round one of the visa procurement ended in total failure.

∼∼∼

Failure to get the visa was not an option, so I contacted the office of our Florida Senator, Andy Crenshaw for help. The Senator's secretary was very cordial and said she would get back to me after speaking with the senator. The next day, she called back.

"Why don't you contact U.S. Congresswoman Karen Thurman?" she suggested. "Karen would be a much better person to contact the U.S. Consulate in Madras, and the Consulate General would then be favorably inclined to issue a visa to your sister. Yours is a genuine case," she added.

That was, indeed, a relief. Without wasting any time, I called Congresswoman Karen Thurman's office and was able to speak with her myself. Karen was very sympathetic to my cause and faxed a letter to the U.S. Consulate in Madras right away. At the same time, I got a second letter from Dr. Najarian, the transplant surgeon in Minnesota, who would be operating on me, and faxed it to Madras. Then I asked Ratnam to fix a second interview and take all the documents, including copies of these faxed messages and try her luck (and mine!) again.

My sister's next visit to the Madras Consulate also turned out to be another ordeal, but this time, the results were in our favor. However, the visa didn't come so easily. Although she was virtually the first one to enter the gates of the consulate and sign in, she was the last one to exit, after a delay of nearly eight hours. They kept her waiting without any explanation, before calling her for the interview. Then came a brutal session of grilling by a female Indian official.

"You know why you are going to America? They will cut out one of your kidneys!" She put it bluntly. My sister never expected such crude language from a government official.

"Are you aware of the complications that can occur for the donor, I guess that's you?" There was sarcasm in her words.

"It is not a piece of cake as you imagine. You should think twice before catching a plane to go to USA."

When she finally took a breath, my sister cut in and spoke: "Madam, I love my brother more than you can ever imagine. I would give him my heart if he needed it. Of course, it is in your hands to issue the visa."

That presumably did it, along with the letters from Congresswoman Karen Thurman and the transplant surgeon. The lady couldn't dissuade Ratnam from her decision, so she relented and stamped the visa in her passport reluctantly. The Consulate General most likely didn't even know what went on behind his back. So much for the consulate's encouragement when somebody is willing to give the "gift of life" to her own flesh and blood! The whole process could have been made easier and less painful if only they could understand what any patient in my situation would be going through. I was somewhat saddened at the prevailing attitude in India regarding live organ donations. In the U.S., everybody is encouraged to become an organ donor. And registering to become a cadaveric donor is quite simple too - just check "yes" on the driver's license application or renewal form. I understand the attitude has changed for the better in recent times and the entire process has become easier now in India.

Ratnam's husband, Aniyan *Chettan*, was eagerly waiting outside and praying all this time, unaware of what was going on. Ratnam called me from a pay phone as soon as she got out of the consulate, giving me the good news. That was the sweetest news I had heard in recent months. A deluge of relief washed over me. Now I was back on track, there was hope! I wanted her to book the flight right away. But as her son, Madhu, would be taking his law academy examinations soon, her trip had to be delayed almost a month, till July 7, 1994.

13

A Short Trip to Minneapolis

June, 1994

By this time, I was steadily getting worse. BUN stayed under control at 35, but creatinine was climbing fast, now close to 7 mg/dl. All my family members in the U.S., most of them physicians, got together and a decision was made to go ahead with transplantation, the sooner the better. This, of course, meant taking a preliminary trip to the hospital in Minneapolis, Minnesota, for a full evaluation and concurrence from the transplant team. I prayed hard that my sister's kidney would match.

University of Minnesota Medical Center (UMMC) has great reputation for live related-donor (LRD) kidney transplants, and many nephrologists highly recommended the center. Dr. John Najarian, one of the pioneers of kidney transplantation, was the director of the program and an outstanding surgeon. His colleagues, Drs. Don Sutherland and John Mattas, also came with glowing recommendations. Since two lives were involved, I wanted the surgery to be done at the best center.

My wife and I caught a flight to Minneapolis and were greeted by

Susheela's niece, Vatsala (we call her *Vatchi)*, and her husband, Rajan, settled in St. Paul, Minnesota. We stayed with them for four days while the tests were being run.

The day after we arrived, we drove to the Transplant Center at the UMMC. Being in unfamiliar territory and because of the construction all around the bridge over the Mississippi River, there was some difficulty negotiating the complex roadways. We finally reached the destination with the help of several helpful locals who were gracious enough to stop and give me directions. An exchange student from Ethiopia waiting for the bus on the roadside and traveling in the same direction was kind enough to come with us in the car and show us the way to the university.

This was more of an exploratory trip, and our appointment wasn't till the next day. We wandered through a cluster of buildings, a maze of corridors, several elevators and offices almost in a daze, awed by the massive complex that handled thousands of patients coming from all corners of the world. We spent some time in the Mayo Building and Phillip Wangensteen Building, the two main areas of the medical center where many outpatient clinics and labs were located. All around, there were masses of people constantly in motion; it was one busy place, for sure.

Finally, we reached the transplant center and Jane Pederson, the smiling secretary, greeted us and introduced us to the transplant coordinator, Mary Rolfe, our contact person here, who talked in detail about the kidney transplant process at UMMC. Since I had numerous phone conversations with her earlier, she knew my background and my understanding of the transplant surgery that I would soon be undergoing. A video presentation of kidney transplantation was scheduled, and we were herded along with a few others who were also in the same boat.

The video was self-explanatory and reassuring, and Mary would say later, the surgery for the recipient was really easy. But she warned me that I would have to take immunosuppressive drugs for the rest of my life to prevent rejection and would need close monitoring for the first several months. To what extent these drugs would bother me, I would only know later. There was nothing more scheduled at the medical center for us that day, so we went to the Minneapolis museum to get a glimpse of the new dinosaur exhibits and then to the Imax theater for a documentary about Antarctic expeditions which was very impressive and enjoyable. It was enough to momentarily take my mind away from what I would soon be going through.

The following day we reported to the Transplant Center at Phillip Wangensteen Building. I had wanted to see both Dr. Najarian and Dr. Connie Manske, the nephrologist who would be in charge of my medical care while in the hospital. When I went to the registration desk, my name was not there on the list! It took some time before they found it and registered me. Once that was accomplished, I was summoned to the lab and a lot of blood was drawn for chemistries, tissue typing and antibody testing.

Most of the afternoon was spent in the waiting room of the nephrologist, since there were many ahead of me. At long last, the nephrology fellow came around, examined me thoroughly and concurred with all the previous findings. Dr. Manske was the next one to show up, and she went over all the details. The main point of our discussion was about the timing of the transplant. I was hoping to postpone it until the following summer. She emphatically said that would be difficult since the creatinine was rising so rapidly and I had already started manifesting symptoms of ESRD!

"You might go into acute renal failure if you get an infection or some other insult. That means emergency dialysis, you know," she warned.

"Oh, really, even though creatinine is only 6.5?" I asked.

"Unfortunately so," Dr. Manske said, as nicely as she could.

I dreaded the possibility of emergency dialysis. As if Dr. Manske was picking up the thread of my thoughts, she added this for good measure: "Don't come here with a catheter hanging from your neck! Infections and other complications occur more often in such settings."

She was emphatic enough in her admonitions for me to receive the clear message.

"We would like to transplant you in early fall," she said.

Thus the decision was made for me.

～～

Later Dr. Manske and I discussed the many medical aspects of IgA Nephropathy and the pros and cons of surgery. One of my main complaints at this time was the constant itching of the skin, most likely from high phosphorus levels in my blood, all too common in ESRD patients and a well known cause of itching. Phosphorus is an essential mineral needed for healthy cell function. It was something difficult to control, but she suggested that a low-phosphorus diet coupled with phosphorus-binding antacids would help. However, I had already tried all these with only limited success.

Finally, Dr. Najarian showed up. An impressive personality, he looked like a football player. Later I found out that he was, indeed, on the football team of UCLA during his college days. His son, Jon Najarian Jr., used to play for the Tampa Bay Buccaneers, our home team in Florida, he told me, and I suddenly remembered seeing him on the TV financial channel CNBC many times. Dr. Najarian examined me and then explained the surgical protocol. He made it seem like a routine surgery, allaying my fears. Though I requested it, he couldn't promise if he would be able to fix my left inguinal hernia at the same time.

By 5.30 p.m., we were out of the building, knowing full well that I still had a long way to go. In any case, at least the ball had started rolling. Everybody involved with my care unanimously agreed that I was now ready for the surgery. The only reason I had wanted to postpone it was to wait until our daughter, Sandra, a senior at Hernando High in Brooksville, graduated from high school and started her six-year BS/MD Honors Program at the University of Miami. Then I would have one less matter to worry about.

"I don't think these kidneys will last that long," Dr. Manske said. "You could be lucky, but I wouldn't bank on it."

Although I consider myself a positive thinker, eager to follow the consultants' expert advice, this was such an important decision, I had to be absolutely certain that the timing was right. Needless to say the idea of taking immunosuppressive medications for the rest of my life was uncomfortable, even scary. "The first three months will be rough," Dr. Reddy had warned me. "But, Ravi, *transplantation* is *the new treatment, this is the cure for your condition*," he emphasized.

～～

Having read Robin Cook's persuasive thriller '*Coma,*' I knew how hard it is to get organs for transplantation and to what extent people may go to procure an organ. Though fictional, the frightening details portray "how a few senior surgeons make sure that patients undergoing even a minor surgery in Boston Memorial Hospital do not wake up. They are kept in a comatose state and remain that way for harvesting the patients' body parts." The plot haunts the reader.

With a suitably matched kidney, one can live comfortably for many years. In spite of having a potential willing donor, here I was still a doubting Thomas!

"I think it's much better to do it now," Susheela repeatedly admonished. "*Kochoppol* is getting older. Right now, she is in good health and perfectly willing to help you. Let us get going. No more dillydallying."

Back in Florida, I had to undergo a few preliminary tests before surgery. First was an exercise stress test with nuclear imaging of the heart for evaluation of any ongoing active coronary heart disease; I passed the test without any difficulty. This was mandatory since I had a coronary angioplasty and stent insertion for unstable angina only a year ago. Because of some minor bowel problems, I also had a thorough gastroenterological examination by Dr. Joseph Caradonna of Tampa and only a tiny colonic polyp was found. I even had a couple of black moles removed from my body by a dermatologist in anticipation of future lifelong immunosuppressive therapy. Some of these moles could turn malignant later on and, immunosuppression is a major risk factor for the development of cancer.

14

THE DAY OF THE MATCH

August 6, 1994

MY SISTER FINALLY arrived at Kennedy Airport, New York, at the scheduled time after a long flight from India. My niece, Mini, a physician in Brooklyn, went to the airport and helped her get on the flight to Tampa, Florida. I eagerly waited outside the arrival terminal of the Delta flight looking at every passenger emerging from the aircraft. I let out a sigh of relief as soon as I saw her smiling face.

Ratnam looked visibly tired after the long journey, first from Kochi to Mumbai by Indian Airlines, then to New York by Air India, covering nearly 7,000 miles and finally, to Tampa. But she was excited and relieved to see me. We collected her baggage and were on our way to Brooksville. I thought this day couldn't come soon enough. She was my lifeline, coming all this way, willingly ready to donate one of her precious organs. I only hoped that she would be a match for me. Her blood group was O positive like mine, which was mandatory for compatibility testing.

Three days after she arrived, there was a strike among the workers in Air India and my nephew, who was scheduled to travel by the same airline, got stranded in Chennai (Madras) for several days. Thank God, Ratnam was able to leave just in time and reach Florida without any hassles.

She underwent all her routine testing within a week after her arrival. I was holding my breath, knowing I couldn't handle the pressure if her lab results turned out to be abnormal, or if she was found unsuitable for transplant for any reason. "Positive thinking, please," I reminded myself for the umpteenth time. But the process was not without some anxious moments. Although her creatinine was normal on two occasions in recent months, the first creatinine clearance on the lab test here came back as only 45, just half of the normal range! But she never had any kidney disease. I pointed out this discrepancy to the lab technician and requested a retesting. Then they found out there was some glitch in the estimation and agreed to repeat it. But we decided to do it in a different lab and the result turned out to be quite normal! Subsequently, she had her IVP (intravenous pyelogram) and other X-rays in the hospital. All turned out to be normal.

So the first hurdle was over!

The next step was to send Ratnam's blood sample to Minneapolis for testing. This is called HLA (Human Leukocyte Antigen) Tissue Typing, a must before any transplant. The success lies in the body being able to accept the transplant without rejection. For this to occur, the donor's HLA antigens should match with the recipient's —at least some of them.

The next day, we all went to Dr. Reddy's office, and blood was drawn in special containers, packed carefully in a styrofoam package and dispatched by Federal Express to Minnesota. I kept my fingers crossed. Within a few days, the eagerly awaited tissue typing results came. Much to my chagrin, we were a *zero match*! For a moment, I was stunned. HLA matching results as per the report looked like this:

Ravindra Nathan
Class 1: A24, B7, Bw60, and Cw7
Class II: DRB1*10, Second DRB*14, DRBeta 3*02
DQB1*501, DQB1*0503

Ratnam Sivaraman:
Class I: A2, A11, BU62 (15), Bu6, BU35
Class II: DQB1 *0601, DRB1 02, DRB*01, DRB5* 01
DRB*13 DRB*0603 DRB*0101

These symbols and numbers were quite alien to me. All I could see was that there were no two numbers the same between my sister and me. Not a single antigen was matching! A zero match! Is that possible? Would they take my sister's kidney now? Do I have to get my other sister here in a hurry as a last resort? That wouldn't be so easy. I didn't know which way to turn.

Susheela was also perplexed at the zero match test results. My sister did share a lot of my facial features, so I thought we would definitely share at least some of the antigens. I called Mary Rolfe for further details, and she referred me to Dr. Arthur Matas, one of the transplant surgeons at UMMC. He didn't appear to be concerned.

"That's no problem at all," he said in a confident tone. "We transplant zero match living related donors all the time. They do much better than even fully matched cadaveric donors. There is better than ninety percent survival for the graft for the first year and probably sixty percent or better survival after ten years." I was dizzy with joy and relief.

"You are very lucky that your cross match is negative. Otherwise, we would have said no," he added. Mary had the same opinion. A positive cross match would mean I had developed antibodies that would react against my donor's organs and their cells. Then I would be non-compatible with my sister's kidney.

Afterwards, the same opinion was voiced by another expert, Dr. Owen Williams from the Harvard Service, whom I consulted over the phone. When I asked Dr. Williams about the timing of the transplant, he said jokingly, "If I were you, I would have had it yesterday!"

That was certainly a very comforting thought. A doctor friend of mine has a brother who is into his 18th year post-transplant and doing well. "At the time of his tissue typing before surgery," my friend said. "We didn't have all these fancy HLAs. It was basically a crude form of testing, but he did all right."

"We still don't know the whole story of HLA typing," Dr. Reddy explained later. "Also, there are many other antigens that may be important and shared by a brother and sister. Some of the recent studies have shown that the best LRD transplants are between siblings. I would have no hesitation, Ravi, if I were you." His voice was confident. Thank God, all the hurdles were over now and the way was clear for us to proceed. Zero match or full match, I didn't have any option, and I decided to get on with the surgery soon.

15

ADAPTING TO MANAGED CARE

September, 1994

MANAGED CARE FEVER was sweeping across the entire U.S. and had become the raging topic for discussion in the media. Hospitals, physicians and patients were all trying to adapt to the new developments in health care delivery. Insurance companies quickly jumped into the fray, wanting to get their share of the medical business.

'Managed Care' was certainly one of the biggest changes to occur in the U.S. healthcare industry thus far. A capitated (discounted) reimbursement plan, as opposed to traditional fee-for-service, was fast becoming the method of payment for services rendered to patients. Under this plan, the physician and institution agree to a fixed annual fee for each patient covered by the health insurance company, a new norm among practitioners and hospitals alike.

As it turned out, managed care in one form or other would become well established later and would provide the greatest opportunity for entrepreneurs and business-savvy physicians. These new economic realities and opportunities led to another concept—health maintenance organizations (HMOs). Soon many large corporations like Well Care, Cigna and Humana came into existence and started negotiating with organizations to provide the health insurance coverage for their employees. They also made deals with physicians for reimbursement of their medical services. All these evolved primarily because of the escalating health care expenditures nationwide.

As a patient going through transplant surgery, postoperative therapies, rehabilitation, and recovery, I received a glimpse of how a prestigious academic institution like University of Minneapolis Medical Center was adapting to the new circumstances and phasing into managed care, practicing state-of-the-art technology and cutting-edge care while simultaneously maintaining cost effectiveness in this highly competitive market.

All of a sudden, the entire nation had become cost conscious, and UMMC followed suit. Soon I found out these changes were applicable to me as a patient as well. When I developed a little post-operative chest pain and cough, I asked if they should do a chest X-ray but the chief resident politely replied, "Your chest is clear on auscultation, we could wait for now." There were no more "routine" EKGs and Arterial Blood Gases, and nurses stopped ordering tests on their own.

One downside of this change in the hospital protocol became evident when I needed an urgent *Doppler* ultrasound evaluation for confirmation of possible clots in the leg veins (deep vein thrombosis.) The chief resident was helpless. He had to summon his superior, the senior surgical fellow, to come, evaluate and concur with the diagnosis, all in the middle of the night, before the test could be ordered! The old hierarchy among the teaching hospital staff, coupled with the new trends in managed care, was being strictly observed.

While I strongly felt that doctors were not the main reason for the skyrocketing health care costs in the U.S., I was happy to see the practice of "defensive medicine" being discouraged even in a high-powered training program such as this, a new trend in the ivory tower of academia. Clinical sense and bedside observations were now given priority and appropriately so. As a clinician, needless to say, I heartily applauded this trend, but as a patient, it was sometimes difficult to accept when they delayed (or didn't do) the tests that were deemed necessary.

~~~

UMMC had a well-functioning day hospital, Masonic Day Hospital that operated from 7:00 a.m. to 7:00 p.m. where many preoperative and other work-ups, including angiography, outpatient chemotherapy, pre-admission physicals, etc. were handled on an out-patient basis. Even the most complicated elective surgery cases were generally admitted only on the day of admission and discharged as soon as the patients were stable. For example an elective nephrectomy patient would be discharged on the fifth day, and an uncomplicated renal transplant patient could go home on the seventh day. The utilization committee was closely monitoring all admissions and discharges.

In the twin city area of Minneapolis/St. Paul, about 70% of medicine was under managed care–more than any other market in the country. A pioneer and world leader in many medical specialties, including cardiac surgery and the entire field of organ transplantation, this tertiary care center also was fast adapting to the financial pressures brought on by the new world order. The Minneapolis market was the most integrated in the nation at that time. Sooner or later, the rest of the country was bound to follow suit.

The positive side of all these reforms was the resurgence of good old clinical medicine practiced at the bedside. Instead of just ordering more tests that may be denied by the HMOs, doctors started listening to patients' complaints more attentively and using their stethoscopes more often to do better clinical evaluations—quite a turnaround in the heavily laboratory-oriented American medicine.

When I was a young medical student in Trivandrum Medical College, India, my attending physicians – from tutors to senior professors – all taught us how to arrive at a clinical diagnosis, using simple but thorough bedside examinations and a few basic tests like chest

X-rays, EKGs, and routine lab work. And most of the time, we arrived at a reasonable diagnosis based on these observations and treated the patients accordingly. They usually got better and went home. We didn't have the fancy ultramodern tests that are available now. However, I must admit, advanced tests are needed for definitive diagnosis, quantification and evaluation of the efficacy of therapy in complex cases, and modern treatments have certainly made a great difference in the survival of patients with serious diseases.

Now fast forward to 2018, managed care in one form or other has become the rule of the land. Large multispecialty group practices are thriving and the future for solo practitioners is growing bleaker. Hospitals are now in the driver's seat, buying up practices. And most physicians, unable to handle the regulatory pressures and dwindling reimbursements from insurance companies, are selling out to the hospitals and becoming their fulltime employees. Meanwhile, the very latest trend of Electronic Health Records, using computers, is becoming the next threat for bedside medicine. The question is, "Have all these measures reduced the cost of medical care?"

I am not so sure.

16

Tragic News on the Eve of Surgery

November, 1994

ONCE ALL MY relatives and I agreed that it was time to go ahead with transplantation. Susheela said in mock jubilation, "Finally, you made the decision, hooray!"

One of my acquaintances in Florida who had a kidney transplant told me, "I'd suffered from chronic renal insufficiency and was debating about a kidney transplant. Then one day I landed in the emergency room with acute renal failure brought on by pneumonia and had to have emergency dialysis." I already knew if some such misfortune happened to me, it would complicate my forthcoming transplant surgery. And Dr. Manske's warning words were ringing in my ears, "Don't come here with a catheter hanging from the neck!"

That was the clincher for me in the end. I contacted Mary Rolfe, my coordinator at UMMC, to get the ball rolling. Since I had a few important engagements pending, I wanted to have the surgery after November 6, 1994. So it was scheduled for November 10, and we planned to leave Brooksville on November 7. I preferred the following week, but Dr. Najarian would be out of the country and I wanted only him to operate on me.

"There is one little detail you need to take care of," Mary reminded me. "You need to get a two-unit transfusion, a unit each from unrelated donors."

The prevailing belief was that pre-transplant blood transfusions will help to prevent rejection and improve graft survival by priming the immune system. (However, this theory has since been disproved and avoiding transfusions whenever possible is now considered state-of-the-art practice!) The transplant could only be done four weeks after the transfusion—which meant, I had to hurry up. But I had some concerns infusing blood from the pooled sources in the blood bank. The horror stories of people contracting AIDS from transfusion had been too frighteningly frequent. I felt sorry for Arthur Ashe, my tennis hero and a world number one in the 70s, who vividly described his ordeal after he contracted AIDS, in his book, *Days of Grace*. Fortunately, by 1994, AIDS antigen screening had become available in all blood banks, so the threat of AIDS transmission had diminished.

Still, not wanting to take any risks, I put out an all-points bulletin to my friends to find out who had O positive blood group and might be able to give me a unit. They took it upon themselves to discuss with their contacts and I didn't have to wait long since three of my friends were O positive and willing donors. Dr. Dawn Augustine, my partner's wife and a pathologist, came to the blood bank with me and gave a unit of blood. Then Dr. Shawkat Kero, a gastroenterologist and a good friend, went on his own in the middle of his busy work schedule and donated blood for me. The samples went to the main lab in Clearwater and I got a call the next day that everything was in order; there was no problem with any antibodies or cross matching.

Finally, I was admitted for a short stay at Bayonet Point Hospital in

Hudson, the adjacent town, for the transfusion after finishing my work for that day—I avoided my regular hospital in Brooksville to maintain some privacy. Dr. Reddy himself started the transfusion and the whole process was over in five hours; I was home before midnight.

On November 5, 1994, I was supposed to chair a symposium, sponsored by the Hernando Chapter of the American Heart Association (AHA), Brooksville. And on November 6, being the chairman for fundraising, I had to participate in a major event for the Hindu Temple of Florida, Tampa. The program was the much anticipated and acclaimed dance drama by the famous troupe of Vempaty Chinna Satyam, a maestro in *Kuchipudi* dance form from India, at the Tampa Bay Performing Arts Center in Tampa. I had to give a ten-minute speech as well on this occasion. A few days before, I had a spell of weakness and hardly thought I could make it through these functions. But determined to keep my chin up and not wanting to give away my specially-guarded secret or draw attention to my illness, I pushed on. Most of my friends still didn't know that I was walking around with renal failure.

By the grace of God, both the programs went well. The AHA symposium was a great success, attracting nearly fifty participants, including many nurses who were always very supportive of my efforts. We raised some of the much-needed funds for the local AHA chapter. The next day's dance performance by the veteran troupe was a sellout, netting a decent profit for the temple. I delivered my lines, a motivational fundraising speech, without missing a beat, fully aware that my BUN was 63, creatinine was 7.1, I was anemic and a full-blown renal failure could be upon me almost any minute!

I was also the editor in charge of a souvenir magazine for the Hindu Temple of Florida that had to be released during this fundraising function. I stretched myself thin trying to fulfill my duties and got 500 copies printed and delivered in time to the Performing Arts Center. Now I felt really ready to take a 'surgery break,' having finished all my assigned responsibilities.

November 6, 1994 will also be remembered for some very sad news in my personal life. Allow me to digress a little here. By the time we reached home after the events, there was a phone call waiting for me. Dipu had called from Boston with the sad news that Dr. Saroja Krishnamurthy (*Saro,* as she was affectionately known*),* my classmate, a dear family friend and a reputed pulmonary physician, had expired at St. Elizabeth Hospital, Newton, Massachusetts. She had been ailing from metastatic cancer and undergoing chemotherapy.

This event struck a blow to my heart, especially on the eve of my transplant surgery. As I was jogging down memory lane, I recalled that at least six of my classmates were now deceased, most of them before hitting fifty. I was puzzled at the irony of fate. Is middle age such a danger zone in our lives? I had also just received some bad news from India. My cousin, Radha *Chechi's* husband, Chandran *Chettan,* only 57, met with a motor vehicle accident and expired at the scene - just prior to his retirement!

"Oh, dear, I need some good news," I told my wife, "especially when I'm going for the big surgery."

"Nothing will happen to you," Susheela reassured me. "We've had our annual quota of bad news. You're going to the best institution and to the very best transplant surgeon. This is as good a preparation as anyone can do; let's have some faith and be optimistic. God will be with us." Well, just the pep talk I needed.

17

<hr />

READY, GET SET...

Nov 7, 1994

WITH ALL MY professional and family obligations over, I packed a suitcase and prepared for the trip to Minneapolis. Dr. Augustine, my partner, agreed to cover for me while I was away and my patients were told I would be on an extended leave for three months. Our 16-year-old daughter was left home in the care of my mother-in-law and *Damumman*, Susheela's uncle, who had just flown from Mumbai for family support. Our gardener came by to clean up the yard and tend the bushes. I strolled over and gave him some instructions regarding his chores of taking care of the tropical plants and trees on our 2 ½ acre lot for the next month.

The day before, I had jogged two miles comfortably and felt good. At least I was in good shape to undergo surgery. Liza Paul, our close friend and neighbor, dropped by and took the three of us, Susheela, Ratnam and I, to Tampa International Airport where we boarded the flight to Minneapolis. The hurricane season being over, there was no big delay at the airport, and the flight was smooth. The weather in Minneapolis was seasonably chilly. While hauling our luggage into the Radisson Inn lobby, adjacent to UMMC, we had a scare when the taxi driver inadvertently tried to take off with our last piece of luggage – a big black bag containing a lot of my everyday necessities! I had no time to go shopping again. It was retrieved just in time with a bit of shouting, a few wild gestures and some sprinting.

～

The next day, both Ratnam and I had to report to Masonic Day Hospital for outpatient workup and Susheela tagged along. The driver of the hospital bus picked us up from the hotel and dropped us at the Masonic Cancer Center, saying that the Day Hospital must be in the same building. Knowing how sprawling this complex is from our summer visit, I presumed he was right.

We got off the bus and started walking amidst all the construction and soon realized our mistake. The Day Hospital had been shifted in its entirety to another area, and it was now in the Mayo Building! Navigating through myriads of labyrinthine pathways, underground passages and a few stairwells, we finally reached the Mayo building, only to be told that Ratnam had to go to the Phillip Wangensteen Building for registration! So we retraced some of the way and sauntered on to that destination. Near the elevator, there was an arrow to Rural Health Clinic Associate Program. Some naughty guy had erased the 'oc' from the 'Associate' and it became 'Ass ate program' – worth a chuckle amidst the tension!' After Ratnam registered, we returned to the Day Hospital for my tests.

Now ensued a long wait. By the time we arrived, after our detours, many others had already signed up. Eons later, a smiling nurse came around, did my blood tests and then asked me to go back to Phillip Wangensteen Building for X-rays and EKGs, which could have been done earlier, if only they had informed me. I didn't know how many more back and forth trips my weak body could handle.

UMMC, indeed, appeared to be an amazing world—an entire

universe within itself, a big, well-oiled, smoothly running machine, serving thousands of patients from all over the world. Many patients, including screaming toddlers and young children, were undergoing tests and treatments simultaneously, a lot of them potential transplant patients too. So many people, so many diseases!

~~~

After the workup, I was given 300 mg of *cyclosporine* in the form of three pills which I gulped down with some water. Although it didn't have a bad taste, the sheer size of the pills bothered me. My immuno-suppression had just started and this would continue for the rest of my life! The thought of being a "changed man" bothered me, but obviously I didn't have any choice. On the verge of a panic attack, I asked Susheela, "Should I or should I not?"

"Don't be silly. It's too late now to doubt anyway," said my exasperated wife.

So I let it be. Alright, I'm ready for the big surgery, come what may.

~~~

The fact that UMMC was one of the best transplant centers filled me with confidence. Mary would later tell me that the entire hospital is so geared toward transplantation that a significant chunk of the hospital income came from this single procedure alone.

They had two transplant divisions - kidney, pancreas, intestines and liver formed one section and, heart and lung formed the other. Both were very active, doing more transplants in their respective areas than many other established centers in the U.S. In addition, UMMC also had the reputation of pioneering a direct, safe approach for open heart surgery in the early 1950s under the leadership of Dr. Clarence Walton Lillehei, considered the 'Father of Open Heart Surgery,' who lived and worked here throughout his entire life. Now they were waiting for their first case of small bowel transplant.

This day would turn out to be an eventful one for Ratnam too. She was told by the transplant group that she must have a full physical examination first. Unable to speak English fluently, she was worried about communicating with the examining physician. Susheela promised to be her personal interpreter. But Ratnam was pleasantly surprised when the surgical resident, Dr. Jyothi Kesha, showed up to do the physical. Jyothi, a very pleasant young lady, originally from our home state Kerala in India, was able to speak fluent *Malayalam*, our mother tongue! My sister was thrilled; she even promised to drop by the doctor's parents' home in Perumbavur, when she returned back to Kerala.

"You look okay, so we'll schedule you for a renal arteriogram tomorrow," Jyothi said. This meant snaking a tiny catheter through the femoral artery into the abdominal aorta, the large artery inside the belly and then injecting a radio-opaque dye to visualize the kidneys and both renal arteries. I jokingly asked Ratnam if she had any second thoughts about the whole procedure, including the looming kidney harvest. In her infinite love and affection, she repeated what she told me earlier in an unwavering voice, "I will give you anything, not just my kidneys, even my heart, if you need it." I had to turn my face, lest she would see my tears.

18

<center>~~~</center>

PRE-OPERATIVE PREPARATIONS

November 9, 1994

ALL OF US reported promptly at 7:00 a.m. to the Transplant Center Evaluation Unit at Masonic Day Hospital. The place was already abuzz with a lot of patients in various stages of testing and treatment. Judy, the nurse in charge of both of us that day, promptly came forward, introduced herself brandishing a needle to poke us and proceeded to take some blood for a few last minute tests including a final cross match. This pre-transplant cross match was the final acid test for me; if by any chance it didn't match, the game would be over in a jiffy and there would be no transplant!

This is a lymphocyte cross match and is done by using my serum and the donor's lymphocytes in the blood. An elaborate process, the pre-transplant cross match required stages of incubation with the addition of an immune material, *complement*. This process detected any anti- HLA antibodies, often called 'panel reactive antibodies (PRA)' in my system, which are directed against the donor's tissues. I already had one done about six weeks earlier and this repeat test was to make sure that I hadn't developed any antibodies in the interim. Patients awaiting transplantation usually have their PRAs checked periodically to allow an ongoing assessment of their chances of a positive cross match. I hoped fervently that this final cross match would be negative, but I would have to wait another twenty-four hours for the result. They wanted it done as close to the surgery as possible.

Now Ratnam was ready to go to Cardiovascular Radiology for her arteriogram. Once again, we went through a myriad of corridors, changed floors a couple of times, got out of the Mayo building and finally reached the UMMC Radiology Department where we were greeted by a second-year radiology resident physician. Later, Dr. Tom Myers, the attending radiologist, would come in and explain everything to us. Dr. Myers looked like the stereotypical erudite physician, sporting a finely trimmed beard and displaying a distinguished demeanor. The resident had to stick Ratnam several times to get the needle into the femoral artery and even then, the blood return from the needle was not smooth and steady. So Dr. Myers took over and easily passed the angio-catheter up the femoral artery and aorta and positioned it at the level of renal arteries. He started injecting the dye via a special power injector. I had already warned Ratnam about the heat wave she would get when the dye, *Renografin*, passes through her system, so she was not alarmed. Having successfully completed the arteriogram, all of us met in the conference room for a review of the images and further discussion. I held my breath and prayed, "No last minute glitches, please."

Dr. Myers pointed at the films on the view box that showed Ratnam's right kidney had two renal arteries, while the left one had a single artery at its origin that quickly bifurcated into two. He therefore felt the left kidney would be more suitable. In order to visualize the area better, he took the additional trouble of getting a Digital Subtraction Angiography, a special fluoroscopy technique that gives sharper images. Later Dr. Najarian's entire resident team was there to review it and reached the consensus that Ratnam's left kidney was more suitable for the transplant. Removal of the left kidney meant they would have to remove the left 12th rib as well, the latter being so close to the left kidney. This would cause some post-operative pain.

I accompanied Ratnam back to the Day Hospital for post-procedure recovery and then went to the admitting for registration. After taking care of a few simple formalities, I was admitted and taken to 5 C, the Transplant Recipient Unit, which would be my home for the next one week. My lunch was reduced to a glass of apple juice, as part of the prescribed liquid diet. "Pre-op precautions, you know," the nurse said in a kindly way. Once admitted, there was an almost never-ending parade of nurses, doctors and paramedics coming in for various purposes. Kathy, a nurse's aide, was the first one to arrive to take my weight. It showed 56.5 kg and I told her that was wrong, since my usual weight is around 61 kg. Shrugging her shoulders, she replied, "We just go by *our* scale."

Nurse Durcell was the next to arrive. She would be my primary transplant nurse and would follow me through surgery and recovery. I had to fill a few more papers. Soon the transplant surgical fellow, Dr. Jacques Pirinni, came by; finally it was the turn of the transplant surgeon and head of the program, Dr. Najarian, who had the most authority and responsibility for the patients. We had a nice chat and he reassured me that everything should go well.

The medical nephrology team showed up next. Dr. Ahmed Nasser, a senior nephrology fellow, examined me briefly; he would oversee any dialysis requirements I may have. I didn't even want to think about dialysis, but if the new kidney didn't immediately work, I might need it. It was comforting to see that all possibilities were being covered. He also reassured me that living related-donor kidneys should start working right away and hopefully, I wouldn't need dialysis. A junior resident from the anesthesia team, Dr. Craig, was the next visitor. He announced somewhat apologetically, "I'm actually from oromaxillary service, presently rotating through anesthesia." That probably meant "Don't ask me too many questions about tomorrow's anesthesia!" and I obliged.

Just as I was getting tired of this procession of visitors, Miss Mary Lundquist showed up. She was the female chaplain and was here to take care of my spiritual necessities. This boosted my confidence; the hospital hadn't left out anything, which was admirable.

"I am still in seminary, two more semesters to go," Mary announced politely. "If you have any religious preferences, please let me know," she added. So I was getting a student, not a fully ordained priest!

"Yes, I do. I am a Hindu, our worship services are quite different," I informed her.

"Now, let me check my book, I believe we have somebody to call on, if we have to," she said and started thumbing through her book, but couldn't find the name of any Hindu priest. We chatted a little bit about spirituality and divinity; I was happy to see she had taken her vocation very seriously. It was my first encounter with a female minister. We uttered a non-denominational prayer together for the success of my sister's and my surgeries.

"Tomorrow is going to be a momentous day in our lives, so please give us your blessings, my Lord," I prayed.

Dr. Paller, the attending from the nephrology department, arrived soon, with Dr. Nasser in tow. We had a lengthy discussion about ESRD. I asked them if they also agreed that the timing was right for my transplant, although it was a moot question now. Dr. Paller enlightened me on the current thinking. HCFA's (Health Care Financing Administration) definition of ESRD is when GFR, the equivalent of creatinine clearance, is down to 10.5 cc/ min. My creatinine clearance would be about there now, taking into consideration my small body frame. So, there was no doubt that the time was right for transplantation.

Once the procession of staff was over, I turned my attention to the patient in the next bed, Jesse, a ten-year-old boy, who looked more like six. His was a poignant story, as told by his young mother. Apparently, both his kidneys had been removed because of *vesicoureteric reflux*, a condition in which urine from the bladder backs up through the ureters and damages the kidneys. Normally, urine flows only downwards from the kidneys into the bladder via the ureters. Most children outgrow this condition with proper treatment that may include surgery as well. Jesse wasn't that lucky, as his condition was not recognized early enough. He was showing some stunting of growth. The mother noticed that there was something wrong when Jesse's younger sister started beating him in games and passing him in height. His bones became weak— a condition called *osteomalacia* or softening of the bones, commonly associated with kidney disease and his growth had become stunted. The mother took him to the family physician and then a kidney specialist. Alas! By this time he was already in kidney failure and had to be admitted to the hospital immediately to have a Hickman catheter put in his neck and started on dialysis. Now he was recovering from bilateral nephrectomy (removal of both kidneys), no small surgery for a little kid.

"As soon as this ordeal is over, he will need a kidney transplant and I am going to be the donor," the mother said beaming with pride. "My little boy is going to be all right," she said looking at Jesse, exuding affection.

I felt sorry for the poor kid, who, at such an early age, had to go through so many tough ordeals. I decided that I should count my blessings rather than complaining about my fate. At least I had come this far.

Feeling a bit tired, I decided to take a nap. But soon Bandy, my new nurse, woke me up. "Is there a shift of nurses every two hours?" I enquired with unmasked irritation.

"Well, Dr. Nathan, you need a *kayexalate* retention enema, your potassium is up," Bandy told me in a matter–of–fact manner.

"How high is it? It was only 5.9 at admission."

"Oh no, it's 6.9," Bandy was adamant even when I showed her my copy of the report. But when I insisted, she relented.

"There must be some confusion here; let me go back and check what's going on," said Bandy and quickly retreated to the nurses' station.

She was a bit unhappy; she wanted to finish the enema and get on with her other chores. I didn't care to go through this ugly stuff and violate my bottom for nothing. Unfortunately, I failed in my mission when Bandy promptly came back and admitted that my potassium was only 5.9, but that was still too high; so I would need the enema and then have the test repeated. As my bad luck would have it, I wound up with not one but two enemas and spent a considerable amount of time on the throne! Bandy trotted off smiling victoriously, having won the battle with an arguing physician.

Durcell came and announced that I had visitors from Florida. Not a minute too soon, I thought. It was Mini (Dr. Sushama Venugopal) and Venu (Dr. C. Venugopal) West Palm Beach, my sister-in-law and her husband—another pediatrician/cardiologist combo in our extended family. They had come all the way to Minneapolis to give the three of us moral support and oversee anything I might need. I felt more confident about the surgery now. Mini looked at the sign board hanging on the wall over my head, studied it for a few seconds and chuckled: "It says here - Dr. Nathan, wife Dr. Nathan, son 3/4 Dr. Nathan….wow, that sure is interesting!" All of us smiled. Durcell, with a flair for humor, had done it; she was referring to my son who was a 4th year medical student at Boston University Medical School, doing an elective rotation at UMMC at this time, to be with me.

A pretty winter scene was on display as I looked out the window. Naked trees lining both sides of the Mississippi River etched in the backdrop of a bluish-gray sky with streaks of pink as the sun went down over a desolate jogging trail, just as in a picture postcard. The outside temperature had dipped to 30°, a far cry from the balmy Brooksville I left a few days ago.

My reverie was interrupted by Sandy, the new night nurse. "*Golytely* time!" she announced cheerfully.

"What?" I asked, puzzled.

"Come on, doc, don't you know? You have to drink all this to clean out your bowels. Tomorrow is your big day, right?"

She held up a bottle of *golytely*, the oral solution given prior to surgery to clean the bowels, which produced severe diarrhea, certainly

SECOND CHANCE

the intended action of the drug. I could see myself dragging in and out of the toilet for the next several hours. After drinking half of the stuff, I felt nauseous and having had copious bowel movements already with the enema, I didn't wish to overdo the evacuation routine. The nurse reluctantly agreed.

~~~

As it turned out, there was only one transplant surgery for the following day – mine. My sister was ready and eager to present me with the ultimate gift. Venu checked the OR schedule, posted in the front lobby with my name for LRK (Live Related Kidney transplant) and possible left inguinal herniorrhaphy. I was glad this was taking place away from home, where all my friends and acquaintances would have been incessantly calling. Here, I was a private citizen, an out-of-state stranger.

19

⚬⚬⚬

To the Operating Room!

November 10, 1994

FINALLY, THE DAY of reckoning! I was awakened by the surgical intern at 5:00 a.m., three hours before surgery. "Problems?" I asked.

"Your potassium is still high at 6.0," the male nurse said. I didn't understand why it was still up in spite of all the interventions the previous night.

"We need to start a glucose and insulin drip now," he added. This was an emergency treatment to correct the problem quickly before surgery. Otherwise, the surgery would have to be postponed, the last thing I wanted.

"Oh, one more thing, you'll need to take these too," he said as an afterthought and gave me six cyclosporine capsules, something I hated at that moment. These smelly 100 mg pills, literally the size of a walnut, weren't exactly my favorite; I had nausea from it the other day, when I took it for the first time. As an additional insult, he proceeded to take some more blood. "For a final cross match," he said as he exited. Both my arms had literally become pin cushions.

Dipu came by to bolster my confidence. Susheela, Venu, Mini and Vatsala, also had arrived. After all the required tests, Ratnam had gone back to the hotel the previous evening, to be admitted very early on the morning of the surgery because insurance rules disallowed an overnight stay for her even though her surgery would start at the same time as mine.

Karen, my new nurse, arrived smiling to take my vitals.

"You need another *hibitane* bath and scrub," she said.

After the one I had last night, I thought I was clean enough for surgery.

"Not so," Karen said. "Need one more. Oh, you will get another chance to see your sister in the anesthesia induction room," she added before she left.

Yes, I liked that. After Karen left, the room was strangely calm. Only the rhythmic sounds of the pneumatic stockings inflating and deflating from the next bed interrupted the silence. A few minutes later, Karen came back to tell me that I would need a Foley catheter, something I abhorred. The memory of the last one at Bayonet Point Hospital following an angioplasty, was fresh in my mind. I had developed a severe urinary infection that gave me much agony for several days.

My transportation arrived promptly at 7:00 a.m., and I was wheeled into the anesthesia induction room while my loving family members held a nervous, prayerful vigil in the waiting room. When my trolley came to rest, I found myself lying next to Ratnam's. They kept the trolleys so close to each other that we could hold hands one more time before the surgery. Then the chaplain called on us for a last minute holy communion with God. I knew the importance of prayers when one is about to enter into a world of uncertainty.

"Lord, please make sure my sister and I come out of this surgery safe. She is doing a great sacrifice for me," I whispered under my breath.

After that, I felt lighter and less anxious. Now it is up to Him, I told myself. After the chaplain left, Ratnam and I gave high fives. Soon we both would be asleep and our bodies would be at the mercy of the surgeons' knives. There was no guarantee about the outcome; one could only hope for the best.

The anesthesiologist came next to explain a few things about surgery and anesthesia induction. Very courteous and comforting, he treated me both as a patient and as a doctor. His words were encouraging. "It's pretty much a standard surgery, and we do this often enough."

That calmed my fragile nerves. I always had the fear of somebody shoving an *endotracheal* tube (ET Tube) down my throat when I am still half awake.

"Don't worry, it won't happen here," he said reassuringly. "I am going to give you some IV sedation first."

My consciousness faded away in a few seconds, carrying me into a blissful oblivion.

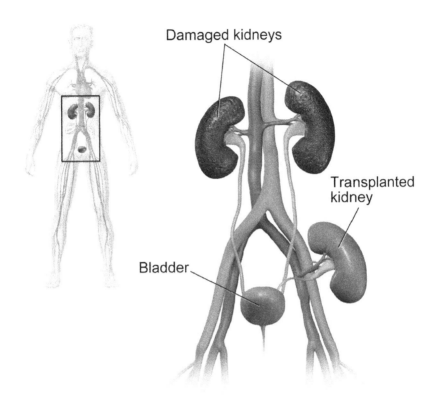

Kidney Transplant

Figure 2: Anatomical diagram of transplanted kidney
(Illustration courtesy of Bruce Blaus, Wikimedia Commons)

PART II
RECOVERY

20

$$\text{\textasciitilde}$$

RECOVERY – OR WAS IT?

November 10, 1994

THE NEXT THING in my memory is of waking up totally confused and disoriented. A lot of people were milling around my bed, eagerly watching my recovery from anesthesia. Many wires and tubes were hanging from my body. Several monitors with the leads hooked on to various body parts were displaying images and emitting a variety of sounds. They covered my vital functions, one measuring the heart rate, another recording the EKG, yet another measuring my breaths and oxygen saturation in blood, the indwelling bladder catheter measuring the urine flow, and more.

There were several doctors, nurses and residents, some in their surgical outfits, keenly observing everything, shouting orders and making remarks to each other. I recognized Dr. Najarian's face in the crowd. He was trying to reassure me that everything went well but I felt a bit agitated, feeling almost like a prisoner. As I became more lucid, I realized the surgery was over and they were overseeing my return to consciousness. The anesthesiologist was trying to wake me up completely before he could leave the area.

I figured it must have been close to five hours or better since I went into the OR. There was a big bandage covering most of my abdomen and upper thigh. My whole belly appeared to be swollen although not very painful. My vision was a bit blurry. I tried to move all my limbs to ensure there was no weakness. Although rare, I had seen patients wake up with stroke and even heart attacks, especially after cardiac surgery. I remember insisting testily to Dr. Najarian that I needed to stand up and stretch. My OR nurse warned me, "Oh no, you can't do that, not yet, you just had surgery. It will disrupt all these lines." In my dazed mind, the only thought I had at that moment was that I must stand up just for a few seconds to make sure my body was intact and I didn't have a stroke. I ignored the panicked expressions on the faces of all the family members.

"No way!" I heard the anesthesiologist shout. I must have made quite a ruckus and created an unpleasant scene because of my stubbornness. Finally, Dr. Najarian relented, and I got my wish. He must have understood my predicament, being a doctor and never having had any previous surgery. All the doctors and nurses together hoisted me from the bed and made me stand up. Hooray! My limbs are moving! But even that assisted movement made me so exhausted I had to lie down right away.

"Your sister is doing fine," my nurse informed me after I gained my composure and was fully awake. The cumulative effects of the sedatives and anesthetics had finally worn off. I felt a little embarrassed that I didn't ask that question first. Was I selfish, worrying about myself first?

Venu told me later that Ratnam had come out of anesthesia without any problem and the first thing she asked was, "How is Ravi?" What an unselfish love! And this, while recovering from her own donor nephrectomy! The surgeon would tell me later her operation was more complex and difficult than hooking up the transplant kidney in my body. We counted our combined blessings.

Finally, I was wheeled out of the recovery room back to my transplant floor, 5C. A small 'reception committee' consisting of Venu, Mini, Susheela and Dipu, was waiting there to greet me, along with my nurses and a few residents. After settling in my bed, I counted the tubes, wires and all other contraptions that surrounded me. A nasal cannula administered oxygen at 2 litres per minute. A nasogastric tube placed in my stomach exited through the nose, connected to the suction machine. This prevented any aspiration, a common problem in the postoperative period since one's swallowing reflexes would be weak and chances of vomiting are high. I was wired to the overhead telemetry unit that monitored my EKG and heart rate. Occasionally, I craned my neck upwards and peeked at the monitor to see if there were any extra beats or ectopics, often a sign of cardiac irritability that can lead to major arrhythmias. None, thank God; my heart was stable.

My neck was hurting a bit, and as I turned to the right, I could see at least three lines coming out of the neck, obviously from the central venous catheter with three portals inserted into my right jugular vein. Otherwise, I would have become a worse pin cushion, my veins being so thin even when well hydrated. And the three lines served me well, one carrying IV D5 Saline for my metabolic necessities that will also flush the new kidney, the second one for IV medicines, especially IV Cyclosporine, the cornerstone of immunosuppressive therapy for kidney transplants, and the third for monitoring central venous pressure, a must for fluid management. Too much fluid could lead to an overload of the circulation, resulting in pulmonary congestion. And too little fluid can lead to dehydration and hypotension that could damage the new graft, resulting in acute renal failure. A *dynamapp* was also attached to my arm for automatic blood pressure monitoring.

Suddenly, I felt a little discomfort in my lower belly and an urge to void, but with the Foley catheter, I didn't have to look for a bottle urgently. And yet the urine flow didn't appear to be as good as it should be. I wondered if the connecting tube from the catheter to the bag was kinked, but the nurse assured me that these painful sensations were bladder spasms and she was kind enough to give me some *ditropan* suppositories to counter them. She reminded me to use the *demerol pump* for pain control as and when needed. This PCP (patient-controlled analgesia) pump is attached to a tube of demerol containing many metered doses and the patient can push the button to get a dose when the pain hits. This capability for self-administration of the drugs saves the patient from calling the nurse every time he or she is in pain. It is programmed to deliver about10mg of demerol in one push and is a godsend for post-operative patients. I didn't want to use it too much, since that can also lead to complications like respiratory depression and aspiration into the lungs.

Both my legs were covered with the special surgical booties that automatically inflated and deflated. And all through the night, the rhythmic sounds of these inflations and deflations of the leg pads kept me awake. As much as I disliked them, I knew they were there for a reason—to prevent phlebitis and clots (DVTs) in the legs, which all postoperative patients were prone to get.

Six hours had passed after the surgery. My mouth, lips and tongue were parched in spite of adequate IV fluids. Even to this day, it is so vivid in my memory. Unable to bear my thirst, I frequently pressed the call button to get some more ice chips. Being still NPO, I wasn't allowed to drink anything. One resident jokingly remarked when he came around to see me that Minneapolis is a dry place and with the heating on during winter, everybody gets dehydrated. The real culprit was the tremendous diuresis from constant IV infusion of fluids given to maintain adequate perfusion of the transplanted kidney, the important first step in preservation of the transplant. Later, the nurses would tell me that my urine volume for the first twenty-four hours was more like ten liters – five times the normal flow!

In spite of all the reassurances, somehow I still felt very uncomfortable. As the night wore on, I could sense that my right leg was getting swollen and stiffer. Although still very groggy from the sedation, in my heart of hearts, I knew there was something wrong somewhere in my body that needed prompt attention. I couldn't express my thoughts properly, but seeing my restlessness and discomfort, Venu came along and looked at my leg and immediately alerted the nurse. She promptly measured the girth of the calf which was only 33.5 cm, but the mid thigh was a whopping 53.5 cm. In a few hours, it was 37 and 57 cms respectively, which meant that the thigh was getting swollen, and there had to be the much-dreaded clots blocking the venous flow!

"Looks like you are developing deep vein thrombosis there! What else could this be?" Venu said with great concern in his voice after examining the part of my legs that could be felt through the wrappings and leg pads and Dipu concurred; Susheela was aghast, knowing its serious implications.

As soon as the nurse conveyed the scary news to the transplant team, there was a stampede of doctors, mostly residents, each one eager to examine me and diagnose the crisis. An unanticipated post-operative complication always created a lot of anxiety. The first-year resident, Dr. Eugene Lee, considered this a hematoma. I wanted Dr. Najarian to be informed pronto but he said that the senior resident and transplant fellow had to see me first, obviously the UMMC's strict hierarchy had to be followed. Dr. Harmon, the senior surgical resident, was befuddled, feeling there definitely was a clot and started me on low dose heparin.

By the time Dr. Pirinni arrived, my entire right leg was swollen and I didn't have any sensation in that leg, especially along the outer side of the thigh. He was quite concerned and realized the urgency of this new conundrum. Panic and disbelief were written all over the faces of my family members. "Now what?" they wondered aloud in immense desperation.

Little did I realize at that time, this was only the beginning of a nightmare that would stretch out for the next several months!

21

BACK TO THE OR!

November 11, 1994

THIS WOULD TURN out to be one of my worst days ever!

It was the morning of the second postoperative day. The right leg showed increasing swelling with pain. There was no measurable improvement with heparin. Now everyone was extremely concerned. After a flurry of discussions, phone calls and frequent evaluation of the status of my leg by residents and nurses, everyone agreed that an urgent Doppler ultrasound of the deep veins in the right lower abdomen, thigh and leg – external iliac, femoral and popliteal veins – was needed to pin the diagnosis and see the extent of the process. Both Venu and I had requested an ultrasound the previous night, but that fell on deaf ears; clearly, no one was convinced then. But now the situation had escalated into a crisis.

Soon I was wheeled into the radiology department. The ultrasound examination, lasting for forty-five minutes, was thorough. The radiology and the surgical residents, along with my family members, were eagerly waiting for the results. The knowledgeable female tech pointed out to everyone the clots in my right leg on the ultrasound images. Indeed my right leg veins were full of clots starting from the popliteal vein at the back of the knee, ascending along the femoral vein in the thigh and extending into the external iliac vein in the lower abdomen where the transplant kidney's vein was hooked up!

This was evidently a very critical matter. The overwhelmed and nervous surgical resident summoned Dr. Najarian stat, but was informed that he was in surgery. However, within an hour, Dr. Najarian showed up at my bedside, radiating vitality. Having seen the ultrasound already, he decided I would need a second surgery. These clots were threatening to impede the blood flow at the site of renal vein hook up, and, if it extended into the renal vein, my new kidney would cease functioning—it was that serious! Not only that, these clots could, at anytime, break off and enter the lung, causing a serious and life-threatening pulmonary embolism. An imminent, possibly fatal threat! All around the world, thousands of people die every year from massive pulmonary embolisms, mostly in the post-operative period. On at least two occasions, I had seen this occur after a major surgery, in my own hospital.

The nervous tension around me was truly palpable, especially on the frightened, drawn faces of my family members. Being a physician worsened the apprehension that came from the knowledge of the dreaded sequelae.

"See what happens when a doctor becomes a patient!" Dr. Najarian commented, to lighten the tension. Doctors and nurses somehow seem to run into all kinds of complications even in the best of hands—at least that is the prevailing belief. Now it became a reality for me. One of my colleagues, a cardiologist who underwent a gall bladder surgery in India while on vacation, developed so many complications that he needed two more surgeries after his return.

"Yours wasn't an easy surgery. I had to literally do an "endarterectomy" on the iliac artery (plaque removal) and then do the anastomosis (surgical connection of the artery of the transplant kidney to the iliac artery)," he said, referring to the widespread atherosclerosis in my arteries.

The anesthesia team was promptly informed, and the resident on call showed up, followed by the attending anesthesiologist. By that time, I was feeling worn out and hoped they would get this surgery over with soon. I felt bitterly disappointed and dejected. After all these elaborate preparations, coming all the way from Brooksville to Minneapolis in search of the best transplant center, I still suffered a major post-operative complication. Obviously, my transplant surgery was different from most of those "easy" ones on record; it had to be special! The ruthless hand of fate was at work again. Susheela's valiant efforts to cover up her mental agony were now futile. Her eyes were puffy from crying. I could sense she was constantly praying to the higher power to somehow get me out of yet another life-threatening crisis safely.

Soon two muscular transport orderlies arrived to take me to the OR again, and lifted me on to the trolley. I couldn't keep my head straight. Two surgeries in two days for a guy who had none ever before! As Hindus, we believe each person is doled out good and bad outcomes based on the *karma* of his previous life. I wondered what kind of sin I had committed in my past life to deserve this punishment. I never got rattled when similar events happened to my own patients in the hospital, but now realized how they felt in such situations. This was my turn; I had to take it in stride and brace up.

～～

The anesthesiologist was waiting for me in the OR. I was prepped and given sedation – *déjà vu!* The induction of anesthesia was smooth. I felt no discomfort and didn't even feel the endotracheal tube going down the throat into my windpipe.

Soon, the knife descended on my belly. Later, the surgical resident explained in graphic detail what went on in the OR. The surgical site was opened and the transplanted kidney along with the venous and arterial hook-ups was examined carefully for any bleeding or clots. It turned out that the site of the new kidney's venous hook-up to the iliac vein was kinked, and there was a large clot extending from this area into the iliac vein downward into the femoral vein and all the way into the popliteal vein—a major catastrophe! The valve inside the external iliac vein had actually kinked into the renal vein, wreaking all this havoc.

Fortunately, Dr. Najarian was able to resect the offending valve in the iliac vein and pull out all those long tubular clots without leaving any residual bits. I shuddered at the thought of what could have happened if one of those clots had broken loose and gone into the lungs! It could be massive enough to block the entire common pulmonary artery or one of its large branches, resulting in instant death! This second surgery lasted two and half hours.

~~~

Sandy, my nurse, truly a godsend, was waiting to attend me when I got back to my room. She explained some of the details and reassured me there would be no further complications. I was still a bit under the effect of anesthesia, but her words did give me some peace of mind. I could see that my thigh was getting smaller, and it certainly didn't feel as tight as before. The uncomfortable bladder spasms started bothering me as soon as I was fully awake, but the surgical resident said the Foley catheter couldn't be removed. For now, I just had to take antispasmodics and helplessly lie supine, so I had to relent.

The edema of the leg subsided appreciably and I felt better during the next two days. I was now on a larger therapeutic dose of heparin for full anticoagulation, not the low dose given earlier for prevention, which meant the possibility of bleeding had to be added to my worry list. I slowly fell asleep listening to the sounds of the pneumatic boots in my legs. The cyclical sounds had a cadence of music that acted like a lullaby in the stillness of the night. Sleep was still very much interrupted. But it was comforting to know that my muscles and veins were constantly being squeezed and emptied and the venous flow going up the thigh was kept intact, preventing any further phlebitis and clot formation. I earnestly prayed there would be no more setbacks and critical care drama.

22

PROGRESS AT LAST!

November 12, 1994

WITH THE NEW diagnosis of 'deep vein thrombosis,' came new restrictions. I was put on bed rest for a few days. Not being able to get up and walk around like other post-op patients was disappointing and lying in bed twenty-four hours a day turned out to be a bigger ordeal than imagined. I had to keep both legs elevated to prevent clots. Then there was the annoying Foley catheter which sometimes leaked and soiled the bed and gave me bladder spasms too. For someone who paid special attention to keeping his body so clean with two showers a day, this was clearly an aberration from the norm and quite upsetting too.

Frankly, I wasn't sure if I would survive these relentless ordeals. Exhaustion oozed from every pore in my body. Stressed out and overwhelmed by a sense of helplessness and desperation, I thought this would be a good time to use the PCA pump to relax and catch some shut-eye. I triggered the button and got a couple of doses of Demerol into me, immediately feeling relaxed. No wonder addicts would go to any extent to procure their drug.

The excessive urine flow continued; I was still making nearly ten liters of urine every twenty-four hours! I wondered if it was too much of a good thing since this fluid loss from the body had to be replaced with constant IV infusion; in fact, they were changing the one-liter bag of fluid every two hours.

"Oh, this is a good thing, Doc. It indicates your kidney is working," the nurse said.

With two surgeries back-to-back and now the phlebitis, I didn't know how long it would take me to recover from this perilous situation.

Reading my negative feelings correctly, Susheela asked me to take a look at Jesse in the next bed. He was recovering from bilateral nephrectomy, and they had started emergency dialysis already. The poor boy was on the transplant list, but would have to wait till he had fully recovered from this surgery. "It's going to be one ordeal after another for him," she gently reminded me. "You shouldn't complain. It could have been worse. Many others aren't even this lucky. You're out of the woods now, and your sister is recovering well. What more can you ask for?"

Well, I got the message and my fears were temporarily assuaged. The words of Rev. Dr. Robert Schuller, the famous preacher from California, came to mind. Addressing a group of Chicago farmers when they were having a poor harvest season and everybody was down in the dumps, he said: "Tough times never last, but tough people do!" By repeating that positive message in my mind, I gradually felt better. It was enough to give me hope and encouragement. I realized one has to weather many storms in life and usually these are transient. If you can somehow survive the crises, life will eventually get back to normal. "Think of all the people in California who have been hit with one natural disaster after another recently," I told myself. First there was the earthquake, next the brush fires, then torrential rains, followed by mud slides – an endless series of miseries! Compared to all those folks, I was definitely better off and should be able to handle these setbacks. So I voiced no further complaints, instead reaffirming the original decision to be tough and somehow get through all these obstacles.

Vatsala and Rajan came to see me that evening. Rajan, a senior manager in a big computer company, is a globetrotter. He just returned from Russia and soon would be going to China and later to India as well.

"Hey, what a good life you are having, Rajan!" I said enviously, prompted by my own wanderlust.

"Are you kidding?" he replied. "I'm not crazy about these frequent travels from one end of the world to the other. I've been doing it for almost twenty years. Right now, I prefer a desk job."

As they say, the grass looks always greener on the other side of the fence.

~~~

It was 9:00 p.m. Sandy brought me a big bowl containing an assortment of tablets and said, "Let's start." It was time to swallow those horse pills again. I placed all the medicines on a clean paper, identified each one to her satisfaction with the correct dosage and then swallowed them while she watched. Sandy and I had to play this game every night. She was making sure of my understanding and compliance with the medicines, critical for my future survival. Indeed, I had a long list of medicines to be taken every single day. The following were the ones just for the night:

Cyclosporine 300mg (3 large pills)

Imuran 175 mg (3 1/2 pills)

Prednisone 15 mg (3 pills)

Zovirax 400 mg (1 pill)

Coumadine 5 mg (1 pill)

Mycelex Troche (1 pill) for swishing in the mouth first and then swallowing.

Maalox (1 pill) to prevent any acidity and heartburn.

I had to repeat this protocol three times a day, taking a similar number of drugs every time. Once, I gagged on the cyclosporine and vomited. But Sandy, a true taskmaster, insisted I take it again.

As the night approached, I became quite restless. My stomach was churning, and I needed something for a few hours of good sleep. Ordinarily, I avoided sedatives. But on this day *ativan* (a mild sedative), came to my rescue. Just as I was dozing off, there was some rustling near the bed that awakened me. It was Andy, the 'line man,' checking on my many IV lines. I didn't know there is a designated line man whose only job was checking the IV lines and ensuring proper function. Being a super specialty tertiary care hospital that dealt with serious and complex surgeries, they had to be meticulous in their approach to patient matters. This is why a person appeared for every little patient-related activity to ensure complete success of the treatment.

As the morning came, the parade started again. First it was Frank, the LPN, to do my vitals. If the blood pressure was high, I got a sublingual *procardia*, a fast-acting antihypertensive. The nurse's aid came next to clean up the room and check on the bathroom supplies. The monitor tech followed; he fiddled with the monitor leads and the CVP line, making sure of a good flow and left only after double checking all the readings for accuracy.

When Daryl came with the breakfast tray, there was a smile on everyone's face. Even the nurses got a share from him. I was on a low-salt, low-fat diet, but they managed to make it palatable enough with a tasty oatmeal porridge, egg-white omlette and a lot of fruits.

By 9:00 a.m., the phlebotomist walked in and announced that he needed some blood. Since the central venous line was intact, it was hassle-free. He took tubes and tubes of blood and walked away triumphant. No wonder I was still anemic! It was Sandy's turn next. She was responsible for administering my drugs and educating me on all aspects of how to maintain my kidney's health. There were so many new things to learn and for a while, I thought I could never get them right. Finally, the fog began to clear, and clarity returned to my mind.

23

THE NEW KIDNEY IS WORKING!

November 13, 1994

THE DOCTORS' MORNING rounds started early. Dr. Lee, the first one to come by, reviewed the bedside charts and lab reports and asked me how I was doing. Did I have any special symptoms that he needed to discuss with his transplant fellow? He left and returned after an hour with his team members, Drs. Pawel Stachowicz and James Harmon, surgical residents, and Dr. Jacques Perrin, the transplant fellow. Of course, they all worked under Dr. Najarian.

Dr. Harmon had done his pathology residency at Boston City Hospital and had now decided to specialize in surgery and transplantation which would take another seven years of training! I admired these people who had the patience and grit to go through such long training programs on modest salaries, to become fine transplant surgeons by the end of the arduous journey. "So you're going to be permanently in training," I joked.

This reminded me of my own long training process, the circuitous route I took before becoming a practicing cardiologist in the USA. After completing my medical school studies (MBBS in India), I did a year of anatomy tutoring, planning to be a future surgeon and my eyes were set on getting the FRCS degree from England. However, on the eve of my travel to UK, one of my advisors, Dr. C. K. Ramachandran, a well-respected physician and Asst. Professor of Medicine, suggested that all good surgeons should have a working knowledge of general internal medicine as well, and I would do well to get some training in medicine first. The clincher came when he went on to say, "It's easier to practice general internal medicine anywhere in the world in comparison to surgery that would require a well equipped operating room, anesthesiologists, surgical assistants and other ancillary services."

After I worked in several medical centers in UK, including University of Cambridge, I decided medicine was the right choice for me and went on to complete my MRCP examination (Member of Royal College of Physicians of London) and then went back to India, at the request of my father and pressure from the Government of Kerala that sponsored me throughout my entire medical studies with a grant. After three years in Kerala Government Service, the wanderlust hit me again, and I immigrated to the U.S. for further studies with my wife of two years, leaving our infant son with his doting grandmother, a heartbreaking decision.

~~~

"Good news!" Dr. Lee said when he returned. "Your creatinine has come down to 2.9. Hopefully, it will drop more," he added enthusiastically. Immensely relieved, I felt like having an instant celebration. This meant my transplant was working well. My little 'baby,' as I called it, must be waking up slowly. I fervently hoped for smooth sailing from here on.

I had heard many horror stories, especially with cadaveric transplants - a 30% chance for acute renal failure post- transplant, during which time the recipient would need dialysis. Even with a living related donor kidney, this could happen, especially with an unanticipated second surgery like mine. But with a good urinary output and decreasing creatinine, I experienced at least a temporary reprieve.

A new patient was wheeled into my room later. It looked like my roommates were changing almost daily. Many of them turned out to be children, since kidney diseases are very common among them and they were all coming here for transplantation. The new guy, John H, a 45-year-old man, had an LRD transplant a year ago. His story was a little unusual. He developed a tumor of the testes, called *seminoma*, about seven years ago, and went into renal failure a year ago, presumably from 'radiation therapy' with *cis-platinum* and other chemotherapeutic agents. His brother gave him a kidney recently. Now he was here with suspected infection from *Cytomegalovirus* (CMV) to which immunosuppressed people like us are more vulnerable.

"All I really need is a shot of some drug, so I can be out of here soon," he said. That would be the antiviral injection, *ganciclovir*, to forestall the progression of his infection. He was pacing up and down the room, calling his friend and berating the delay in getting the treatment started. Later when I enquired what was going on in his life, he unloaded all his stresses on me. His wife left him a year after the transplant. She obviously couldn't handle the new life of round-the-clock medications, thrice weekly blood tests, dietary restrictions and constant vigil. I knew that wouldn't happen to me. Susheela understood my situation well and, as my devoted physician wife, would do anything for me at any time. "We're in this together. Don't worry," she would say often. As soon as the nurse gave John the shot, he scooted out of the floor in a hurry.

～～～

The anesthesia team, including Dr. Carl Newmann, the resident, and Dr. David Pizzuto, the attending, came around to check me. They were happy with my progress so far and told me that I had received three units of packed cells altogether during the surgery. The next to arrive was Dr. David Dunn, the surgical infectious diseases (ID) specialist, specially appointed by Dr. Najarian. We briefly talked about my travails and hoped that I had seen the last of them.

By the time the entire medical crew finished their evening rounds and left the floor, I was feeling hungry, so the arrival of the dinner tray was a welcome sight. It was bass with fried rice, cream pudding, cottage cheese and skim milk. What cream pudding was doing in my low-fat diet menu, was a mystery. But I sampled a bit of everything and felt good afterwards. Next, Lori from Respiratory Therapy (RT) came to check my oxygen line. She was there the night before to do my EKG as well, when I complained of a little chest pain. "We are very versatile, you know," she said with a smile.

At 6.50 p.m., Marcie, my new nurse, asked me to get up and out of the bed. I thought maybe she wanted to make the bed with clean linen. But she announced, "We are going for a trip today."

"Where to?" I asked. I just had my dinner and felt like resting a bit.

"Visiting your sister. Don't you want to see the lovely lady who gave you the precious gift?"

"Wonderful!" I said with a big smile on my face. It had been three days since I'd seen her. I took baby steps to room 515; for a moment, I was overwhelmed with emotion – "Here's my savior!" I said aloud with a galloping heart. She was recovering nicely, but had a bout of mild urinary tract infection (UTI) from *pseudomonas aeruginosa*, a common bug, and was being treated with antibiotics.

I gently squeezed her hand and said excitedly, "We did it, *Kochoppol*, we did it!"

She looked at me with loving eyes and unalloyed joy, and said, "Yes, Ravi. So nice to see you walking. God is always with us."

~~~

Even this short trip to another room was tiresome, so I returned to my room to rest. On my way back, I saw quite a number of sick children, most of them in different stages of transplantation. Some were for kidney, others for liver! It was more like a pediatric floor, with a child in the lap of some of the nurses – either being fed or comforted. Many kids were moon-faced from the large doses of steroids they were taking. Others were pushing their strollers around and chattering incessantly. And the rest were whimpering from the discomfort of a recent surgery.

There was a little boy, Jason, suffering from *oxalosis,* waiting for his transplant. Oxalosis or *hyperoxaluria* is a rare condition where too much oxalate is present in the urine. Since oxalate and calcium are continuously excreted by the kidneys into the urine, both will combine to form calcium oxalate crystals and grow into a kidney stone. Although kidney stones are more common in adults, this poor kid developed calcium oxalate stones in both kidneys that resulted in kidney failure. Little Jason was playful, making himself quite at home. Sometimes he preferred to be in the playpen, sometimes in the nurses' laps, being cuddled. At other times, Jason simply wanted to lie down on the bare cold floor.

This was truly an amazing world – a world of liver, kidney and pancreatic transplants, and they were starting small bowel transplant as well. Patients came from all over the U.S. and other countries as well, including South America and Asia as this was the most acclaimed center in the U.S., if not in the world, for transplants. I felt happy to have received my treatment here.

24

STEADY PROGRESS

November 14, 1994

THE TEAM OF Lou Wenchell, Eugene Lee and Pawel Stachowich, doctors in charge of my care, arrived bright and early. The wound was inspected; it was healing well—thank God, no infection so far. Everyone knew two surgeries back-to-back along with high dose immunosuppressive therapy, can wreak havoc on wound healing. Lou agreed to take the Foley catheter out, much to my relief; it had been bugging me to no end. Another bonus came later – I was allowed to shower. So I quickly shaved, took a nice hot shower and put on some new clothes. Looking in the mirror, I was happy to see my old self. I felt cheerful when Don, the chaplain, called on me. We had a nice conversation about spirituality and our respective faiths.

I hadn't fully realized the extent of the teamwork involved in the completion of a successful transplant before. There were so many groups of people working in total synchrony. Before surgery, the transplant coordinators – there are four of them here, with Mary as my personal coordinator – attend to every detail. Mary was almost the cornerstone of my edifice. The labs play an active role running frequent tests, including special ones like tissue-typing and cross-matching. Once admitted, the charge nurse and the residents are in control, and they orchestrate the whole program quite well. Everything goes like clock-work, nothing left to chance; that's the secret of their success.

A number of non-clinical staff members, also interested in my progress, visited me today. First on the scene was Cheryl, the social worker, who was evaluating my insurance status and making sure that I was not in any way inconvenienced by lack of funds, a very noble thought indeed. "Now that you have a transplant, you are eligible for Medicare," she said. That was very comforting. "At least it will be in effect for three years and will cover all the costly anti-rejection medicines. These are essential to prevent rejection of the transplant, more common in the first few months. Your regular prescription plan will take care of the rest. The transplant team wants to make sure that every patient has access to a steady supply of medications. In the early phase, you can't afford to miss even one dose for fear of rejection."

Ben Newsman, a solemn-looking guy in charge of the utilization review, was the next one to show up. His job was to make sure that patients do not overstay in the hospital and cost the insurance company additional expenses. He said that I was allowed only seven days in the hospital for the transplant, which would be extended by two more days because of the second surgery. "We want to ensure proper utilization of services and oversee that there is no waste anywhere," he explained. "This is an HMO hospital, and everything here is strictly monitored and all rules adhered to." After the visitors left, I decided to take a walk; until now, I had been simply lazing in the bed. But feeling pretty weak when I started walking, I returned to my room quickly.

Andrea, the new nurse, informed me that the doctors were coming for rounds again. The rounds were short and sweet; I was obviously getting better. As soon as they left, Andrea came back, asking me to review the videotape of the transplantation program and drug regimen

I would have to follow. Feeling exhausted, I requested her to postpone it. Sometimes I would get this extreme fatigue and lassitude and would lose interest in everything. I told her the dryness in my mouth was back again. "You'd better drink more fluids," she cautioned gently.

Later, Dipu came by to cheer me up. He was rounding with the Infectious Diseases team and saw a few cases of AIDS. He was now the pillar of my support group since Venu and Mini had returned to Florida.

25

∿

So Far, So Good!

Nov 16, 1994

IT WAS THE fifth day after the second surgery. Why did I feel so worn out? My appetite was back, and I was supposedly recovering well. The previous night hadn't been easy though, I had to go to the bathroom every two hours.

Durcel came in early, although I expected her only in the afternoon. I completed a couple of rounds of walking on the 5th floor, strolling along the corridors, trying to gain strength. When I complained that I wasn't getting better any faster, Durcel said, "Oh, you are doing okay. Our pancreatic [transplant] patients have it much worse, you know. Their surgery itself is difficult, then the complications – abscesses, fistulae.... the healing is so slow. Their post-op monitoring protocol is almost endless." Every day, like clockwork, she would come and reaffirm that I was much better off. Well, that put an end to my whining.

I spotted Tausier, my CNA (certified nursing assistant), stocking up the supply cabinet with the bathroom supplies and other necessities.

She was from Eritrea, a small African country, torn by war and famine. She said the war had ended now, and she could go back if she wanted to, but she was planning to stay, now that her family was here. Her only complaint was the bitter cold in Minnesota - tough to adjust if you were coming from the tropics. How well I knew this, having to face the same problem of adjustment when I first went to London in 1965 from tropical Kerala, and later arrived in New York in 1972.

Susheela brought tea and some goodies for both of us. Later Dipu also joined us since he had to see a consult in the transplant unit. Infectious Disease people always got perturbed when they saw fever in a transplant patient, thinking of all the exotic diseases they are susceptible to. I was happy that my temperature had been fine—at least for the moment. Earlier, there was a hint of urinary infection when I developed some pain while voiding soon after the Foley was taken out, but all the cultures came back negative.

Dipu laid out his plans for the future. He was actively searching for a medical residency position, his eyes set on some good institutions. Afterwards, he would consider doing a fellowship in Cardiology, possibly. But he didn't want to be a perennial resident like some of the others who go for further specialization and research. "I want to earn some money, Dad, before this healthcare system collapses!" he said one day with a smile. I told him that reform or no reform, the American health care system is still the world's best and it was not going to collapse anytime soon. In spite of the invasion from lawyers, managed care bureaucrats, insurance companies and governmental agencies, medicine is still one of the best professions, I reminded him. He knew it and our daughter, Sandra, was also planning to be a physician. I felt good about both our children following the footsteps of their parents.

26

~∾~

GETTING READY FOR DISCHARGE

November 27, 1994

MY CREATININE WAS still like a yo-yo. On the second day of the first surgery, it had dropped to 3.1 (from 6.4) after the intense IV and oral fluid therapy as well as Lasix, a diuretic, the strategy working well. The creatinine and BUN steadily came down, and I felt relieved, but the unfortunate and unexpected setback of DVT and subsequent second surgery did impede the recovery process significantly. The jump in the creatinine to 3.3 made me anxious, as I feared the worst. The residents said I was having a mild form of ATN (acute tubular necrosis – acute injury to kidney resulting in sudden decline in kidney function), but that as long as the kidneys were working, there was nothing to worry about. From my experience of treating many such patients in my own practice, I knew the recovery could take a few days. Some might even need dialysis to tide over during the crisis. I was yet in the polyuric phase, making large quantities of urine. Still it was better than oliguria (not enough urine), which is not a good sign as it reflects diminishing function of the transplanted kidney. If anuria (no urine) sets in, dialysis would be mandatory.

Dr. Lee was in charge of tracking my creatinine and putting it on the bulletin board daily. Seeing it fall to 3.1 was comforting, and two days later, it was down to 2.9. Sandy remarked that this might be my baseline creatinine and not to worry too much. I slept a little better that night.

~~~

The next day, breakfast tray came early and I enjoyed every bit of it as my appetite was great. But what thrilled me most was my new creatinine level– it had come down to 2.7. So, the transplant had started working well! To give Ratnam the good news, I ambled to her room dragging the IV pole - an exhausting five-minute trip. Susheela was also there. Together, we savored the good news. Now I could relax a little. We had a morning counseling and educational session, under the direction of Marsha Zuckerman, the social worker. One good thing here, I noted, was their constant effort to educate and update you regarding the new organ just received and how to take care of it. A consummate teacher, Marsha was really good at explaining all aspects of the post-transplant care. "Overnight, you become a different person, and there is a lot to learn," she said. I was somewhat overwhelmed with all the details, everything from dosage and administration of drugs to filing for Medicare and supplemental insurance. This, after being a physician for thirty years!

An interesting person I met during this meeting was Chuck White. A man in his late 50s, Chuck had a cadaveric transplant about ten years before, at the UMMC and was doing admirably well. He had become a local spokesperson-cum-advocate for transplant patients and was collecting money for the transplant athletes to go abroad and compete. Chuck reassured me that once the immediate post-operative phase was over I should be very active and should get back to tennis and jogging whenever I was ready and felt up to it. Nothing would please me more than getting back to my routines. "I will be in

Clearwater in January. Why don't you give me a call? Maybe we can get together and chat."

Chuck was also quite knowledgeable about tissue matching and rejection. When told that my sister and I was a zero match, he quickly remarked, "A living related donor is always better than a cadaveric transplant; lucky you! There are fifty or more antigens that siblings share which are not in the current testing panel. So relax, you can't do badly." I liked his optimism, and his contagious confidence. Needless to say, this was extremely reassuring.

<center>~~~</center>

The long session I had with Marsha, was very helpful. She explained in detail the names and actions of each drug, how to take them and what to do if I accidentally missed a dose. "When you take *Acyclovir* and *TMP-SMX* (trimethoprin-sulphamethoxazole), you need to flush the kidneys with lots of water. *Prednisone* is another drug to watch for. It increases appetite, but don't simply put food in the mouth impulsively when you feel like it; you'll only get fat. Some people will have an inadvertent hand-to-mouth motion, so-called 'prednisone munchies,' which is no good," she said.

"No chance of me getting fat, Marsha," I said. "All my life, I have been trying to put on a little weight, so I won't look this thin. Maybe prednisone is my answer," I joked.

Marsha smiled and added as an afterthought, "I don't have to tell you contact sports and sun exposure are also forbidden for a while."

"Don't worry about contact sports. I am not into football or wrestling. But do tell me how to avoid sun exposure in Florida?" I said.

Marsha also talked about my going home, which could be scary at first after being under close supervision by the efficient staff. She patiently explained the process of filing for Medicare, which was going to be my primary insurance for the next three years. My current insurance company, Prudential, would become the supplemental. This was happy news, since I knew my 'Minnesota experience' would be costly, to say the least. Toward the end, Marsha reminded me that there would be one more teaching session before my discharge, which was indeed welcome; so much was crammed into my head in one day, I was beginning to forget some of it already.

During our last session, Marsha mentioned that my primary renal care would now be handled by UMMC, with my local kidney doctor as the coordinator-cum-local guardian, so to speak. We briefly discussed the signs and symptoms of rejection and what to watch for. The first three months would be crucial, then it might get a little easier. Rejection was often treatable and controllable, especially the acute rejection process. She warned me never to stop the drugs at any time, since this would lead to rejection, sooner or later. Also I should look for certain signs of rejection like fever, sudden fluctuations of BP, as well as an increase in the serum potassium or creatinine.

I sincerely hoped I would go through the first three months of transplant without infection or rejection. A lot of self-discipline was needed along with positive thinking. I kept reminding myself that this transplant was too precious, and I was the only one who could protect it.

27

AN EMOTIONAL DAY
FOR MY DONOR

Nov 17, 1994

WE HAD ANOTHER teaching session at the main learning center, this time with all the audio visual aids and other paraphernalia. I was wheeled into the Mayo Building where I met several other transplant recipients, including one who had a combined kidney-pancreas transplant. We went over the drugs again. The post-op and long term follow up care was the main topic of discussion. We were also taught how to adjust cyclosporine dosage according to its blood level, using different strengths of the drug and a simple calculation. Also discussed was tapering the dose of Imuran and prednisone, once the kidney function became stable in the next few weeks.

Pandy, our teacher, was superb and guided us through all these calculations. I felt like a child learning mathematics for the first time. She gave us questions like, "If you take 125 mg Imuran, how many pills would that be?" The answer was 2.5 pills, since Imuran comes in 50 mg tabs. I felt silly blurting out many of the answers and noticed funny looks from the other patients in the room, as if they were asking, "Are you a doctor?" I decided to keep my mouth shut, not wanting to look like a show off.

Pandy also suggested that we should check the blood cyclosporine levels periodically since higher levels of cyclosporine (above therapeutic range) can produce renal toxicity, some of the symptoms of which can mimic rejection. So I asked Pandy, "How do you distinguish kidney rejection from *Cyclosporine* toxicity?"

"That is really a very difficult thing," was the answer. Even on a microscopic examination of a biopsy specimen (histology), the transplanted kidney may look normal. But a sudden rise in serum potassium with higher levels of Cyclosporine would tell us if the diagnosis is Cyclosporine toxicity or not. She also gave me some points for prevention of infection, such as frequent cleansing of the hands, avoiding contact with patients who harbor any harmful germs, paying attention to early signs of infection and taking immediate steps for proper work-up and treatment. We were told to call the Transplant Center if we ever developed a fever.

The next discussion was on my follow-up monitoring with serial labs after returning home. A major worry for me was that I would be almost 1,500 miles away from Minneapolis. But Dr. Najarian said later, "Oh, you are just three hours away by air from the Transplant Center, so why get nervous?"

I knew this was 'separation anxiety' as I was about to sever my umbilical cord with UMMC. But it was time to accept that I was a free man with some limitations; yes, I was also thrilled that I wouldn't need any dialysis as long as I take care of my new kidney well.

"There are routine lab protocols for the first three months, tests to be performed at least three times weekly," said Pandy. This included hemoglobin and WBC count as well as kidney function panel that consisted of serum electrolytes, magnesium, phosphorous and calcium.

I told her, at this rate, I might run out of blood! They gave me a lot of CSA (cyclosporine) mailers for sending the blood samples for measurement of CSA levels that would be done at the UMMC. Any changes in therapy would be made by the Transplant Center only.

There was other advice too, already printed in the transplant book, but reemphasized by Pandy for our benefit. "Keep your legs up when you sit; walk around every thirty minutes, no jogging or tennis for six months and remember to inform the Transplant Center of any change in your clinical condition."

When I returned to my room, Susheela was waiting for me, looking flustered. Apparently, Ratnam had become very emotionally upset and started crying aloud for no obvious reason. I went over to comfort her. My sister, who had been a real trooper till now, was hysterical, demanding to see our long-departed parents right away. She was not hurting anywhere and yet was inconsolable, wailing like a baby. Poor Ratnam was both in the real world and in her own imaginary world at the same time. "I can't stop crying, Ravi," she said between her sobs.

"But why? Your surgery is over and you came through with flying colors. The wound is practically healed and your other kidney is working well."

"I just don't know. The whole thing was a bit too much," she said. "But don't you worry, I'll be okay" she added. After her tears subsided Ratnam told us she was very happy that she did her duty and not even for one moment regretted it.

Later, Mary Rolfe explained that some donors go through this temporary "grieving process" at the loss of one of their organs, a part of their own body, as though they have lost a child and may become overly sentimental. But after she gained her composure, Ratnam said, "No, it was certainly not the feeling of losing a part of my body that made me cry. It was the experience of having come through this big ordeal successfully….maybe it triggered an extreme reaction in me." Although Mary Rolfe may have a point regarding the general behavior of a donor immediately after surgery, Ratnam emphasized that she "never ever felt that way even subconsciously." And I believed her.

Ratnam also disliked the food here, the typical bland, hospital diet, even though nutritious. "Oh, how I would love some of our food, like *rice kanji (porridge), pappadam and mango pickle,* may be a little *sambar too!*" These are the standard *Malayali* fare we're used to. Susheela requested Vatsala to cook some of these special dishes at home and bring her some soon after discharge.

Finally, it was time for Ratnam's discharge. She didn't have any special instructions to follow, just to watch the BP and if it went up, start appropriate medications. Her surgical wound was already healing well. She was seated in a wheelchair and I accompanied her to the lobby. But there was one more hurdle to cross. Once again, flooded with inexplicable emotions, Ratnam insisted she was unable to walk beyond the entrance of the lobby toward the van to the Radisson Hotel! So we had to wait for a special van with wheel chair access and I literally froze in the wintry draft whenever the door opened.

But the waiting turned out to be interesting. We were treated to a special sight, albeit a little unglamorous—a big commotion caused by a middle-aged lady. She was obviously a post-operative patient with multiple lines dangling from her body. She had darted out of the Phillip Wangensteen Building with an exasperated nurse hot on her heels trying to control her abrupt movements so no harm would befall her. The patient appeared to be pretty sick and obviously was in one of her foul moods, cussing everybody including UMMC, for not allowing her to smoke in her room! At last, she was allowed to go on the walkway just outside the lobby where she merrily smoked her cigarette in full view of a hundred onlookers. She had a sense of great accomplishment, having challenged this big old institution and won!

While sitting there, I looked around and again realized how big the UMMC complex was. The Phillip Wangensteen Building was a mammoth structure with numerous outpatient clinics. Then there was the Mayo Building, Masonic Cancer Center, Children's Hospital and the huge Medical School building. The whole setup was like a big city mall with shops, eateries and boutiques, masses of people from all over the world moving around, creating a world within a world—one of pain, suffering, hope and redemption. I came here somewhat depressed and anxious, not knowing how it was all going to turn out, but felt so relieved and happy to head back home after the successful transplantation.

I was truly given a second chance—a new lease on life!

28

FINALLY, TIME TO GO HOME!

Friday, November 18, 1994

NOW THAT RATNAM was back in the hotel room where a very compassionate Vatsala kept her company, I hoped she would get some rest and Susheela would have to attend only to me. I was getting stronger, although my BP still fluctuated. Sudden surges in systolic BP can bring on problems like headaches and even stroke or heart failure, so it was a bit unsettling.

My nurse, Lucy, took my vital signs often and reported them to the nurse-in-charge. At times Gale, the chief nurse, would come in saying, "Oh, your BP has gone up to 168/92. Here, take this sublingual *Procardia*." That would bring down the BP to about 140/85. Gale's husband was in the surgical oncology residency program here. She tested me on the drugs I was on, the list being quite long and daunting for any patient. Even as a doctor, I had a tough time remembering the new names, doses and the timings. The list contained the following medicines:

Cyclosporine: 225 mg twice daily after meals

Prednisone: 15mg three times daily after meals

Imuran: 75 mg twice daily – morning and bedtime

Bactrim DS: 1 daily

Procardia XL: 30 mg twice daily but may increase to a total of 90 mg daily if needed.

Acyclovir (Zovirax): 400 mg capsules twice daily

Mycelex Troche: 1 four times daily to ward off any fungal infections.

Maalox: 1 tablespoon four times daily to prevent hyperacidity and emergence of peptic ulcer.

Coumadine: 5 mg daily with monthly blood tests and dose adjustment accordingly.

"At this rate, I won't be needing any meals," I joked. And the lunch they brought was spaghetti and meatballs. Since I had stopped eating red meat altogether, I asked them to bring plain spaghetti with a little marinara sauce over it. Anyway, Susheela had brought a homemade soup and we enjoyed the lunch together. My appetite was gradually coming back. In the afternoon, Carol, my new nurse, came to visit me with the latest test results. The creatinine was still hovering around 3.1.

"Don't worry," she tried to reassure me, looking at my crumpled face. I presumed it was going to take longer for the new kidney to settle down and start functioning optimally. I could only hope the renal function would return to near normal levels eventually.

Dr. Najarian came to see me later. We had a photo taken together and briefly talked about my right leg, which was still a bit swollen. Also, I had a lot of tingling and numbness (paraesthesiae) in that leg. He thought the leg should heal fine, and at this point, there was no cause for alarm. He was flying to Los Angeles to attend a transplantation conference and wouldn't be back before my discharge. But I could catch a flight to Florida any time after discharge the following day. He was always very pleasant with a casual demeanor, both admirable qualities for a surgeon. But we all knew he was one of the most outstanding kidney transplant surgeons in the world. That was why patients from all continents flocked to Minneapolis for this special surgery.

Now that I had the whole room to myself, I felt like it was my own rented apartment and I wished to keep it spotless. Scott, my cleaning man, obliged. Later I took a walk around the entire 5C and 5D without any problem and made it back to my room safely. My strength was improving.

When I switched on the TV, it was all about Hurricane Gordon, ripping through Brooksville and the surrounding areas. "Oh my God, my sleepy town is on the national news!" I exclaimed to myself. Worrying about our house, I called my daughter who assured me it was intact, no trees had fallen, the lawn was getting a good soaking and it should look greener than before; so far, the roof was intact without any leaks. Four days of rain squalls and so far no fatalities or power outages in Brooksville. Hallelujah!

~~~

Saturday, November 19, 1994

Finally, the day of my discharge arrived. I was awake at the crack of dawn. By 7.30 a.m., the first two medical rounds were over. Dr. Lee, who had made a lightning trip to Los Angeles to be with his mother during her surgery was now back, and briefly examined me reviewing the instructions again. Then the entire transplant team stopped by, wished me good luck, and answered all my questions.

Dr. Louise Wentschell's entourage was the next to arrive, giving me the final instructions, especially regarding the post-operative care once I reached home. They felt the creatinine would come down from 3.1 to near normal in due course. The unit secretary, Hatley, at my request, pulled all my reports from the computer including discharge summary, operative reports and lab data. It looked like a tome! Since I had some more time on my hands before discharge, I walked around to check out the layout of the floor and socialize with other patients.

Today, a student nurse was also assigned to take care of me. Crista looked vibrant and eager to learn about my illness, surgery and the implications of having a new organ in my body. She was a little apprehensive when she realized I was a physician, but I allayed her fears by giving her a nice insight into my past and current problems. She wanted to be an RN and was already enrolled in a four– year program.

The transplant station was a mini-city all by itself, quite unique, with a lot of bodies in constant motion. The triangular nursing station was always busy with doctors and nurses and several paramedics constantly milling around. The equipment in patient rooms were buzzing away, emitting all kinds of sounds and flashes of wavy lines coming from the overhead monitors. Yes, medical technology was in full display. Altogether, it was a fascinating atmosphere, maybe a tad alien to a non-medical person.

A few more formalities had to be completed. Durcel came to instruct me one last time about the dos and don'ts after transplant. He went over the drug list and lab protocols again. Didn't I know this by heart now? *Imuran* should always be taken at night as a single dose. *Cyclosporine* should be taken if at all possible at exactly 9:00 a.m. and 9:00 p.m. daily and the level drawn fifteen minutes before the last dose. WBC count has to be kept within 4000 to 11000/dl. If creatinine is more than 3.0, use *Alternagel* for antacid. It is aluminum hydroxide and is used to reduce build up of phosphate levels in people with kidney disease. *Acyclovir* prevents CMV virus, EB Virus, chicken pox and genital Herpes. Nice to know that I was protected in many ways! Needless to say, I was very impressed with how they handled their transplant patients—with tender loving care.

Marsha, my social service worker, had already called Chronimed Pharmacy, a nationwide chain that supplied the drugs for transplant patients. I would be on anti-rejection medications for the rest of my life. Marsha phoned them the day before and the drugs were supposed to arrive before lunch. They had already given me a tracking number, just in case.

By lunch time, I was getting a little anxious about the drug package and was about to call them. Right then, Hatley, our ward clerk, walked in and asked me if I was expecting a parcel from Chronimed. The parcel was left at the front lobby with my name on it but it didn't quite make the short trip to 5C! Hatley was kind enough to pick it up for me.

Finally, after ten days of hospital stay, I was ready to go home. As per hospital policy, I had to be taken by a wheelchair to the lobby. It was a cool day, and I was already thinking of my immune-suppressed status that made me vulnerable for infection when exposed to cold weather. Susheela had called the hospital escort van to take us to our hotel. By the time we were down in the lobby, the van was already pulling in, and we reached the Radisson in less than five minutes.

～～

I had a comfortable night in the hotel room. Thanks to the generosity of Vatsala and Rajan, there was no dearth for good Indian food. The four of us, Susheela, Ratnam, Dipu and I, were huddled together in a double room. Dipu would stay with us until we left for Florida the following day. Then he planned to stay in a rented apartment for three more weeks to complete his rotation in Minneapolis.

Ratnam, however, was still having a rough time. She continued to be a bit anxious and tense. Although she had completely recovered from her surgery, she looked weak, often emotional and occasionally tearful. She was content to sit by herself and read from our scriptures *Bhagavad Gita* and *Bhagavatham;* occasionally she needed some assistance for showers and dressing. We tried to comfort and counsel her as much as possible and hoped she would cheer up soon. I surmised that subconsciously, she may still be grieving for her lost organ. But at the same time I thought I was wrong because she had taken it as her sacred mission to save me from my illness by giving this precious gift.

A sister's love for which I will forever be indebted.

～～

The Radisson Hotel turned out to be a nice, cozy place with all the basic amenities. So close to the hospital, it was a big boon for us. They also had a 'Kidney House' that accommodated the relatives of the renal patients. UMMC knew how to offer the ultimate care to their patients and family members.

29

MORE SETBACKS AT HOME

November 21, 1994

OVERNIGHT, IT TURNED very chilly and started snowing in Minneapolis. Our flight to Tampa, Florida, was scheduled for the morning and my anxiety kicked up again, this time about the possibility of delay at the airport or even cancellation of the flight. The cab took us along the Mississippi River, the scenic route lined with elms and maples, quaint cottages and small buildings. The trees were naked and appeared as wavy lines etched in the backdrop of a gray cloudy sky with a baleful look—typical of a Midwestern winter.

Thankfully, the flight was on time. It was cold even inside the airport, and I worried about catching an infection in my new immuno-suppressed status. At the Tampa Airport, the smiling faces of Liza and Paul greeted us. There were two wheelchairs at the gate, and Paul thought that these were meant for us, the two patients from Minneapolis. But when he saw us walking out the gate, he was surprised. "We don't need any wheelchairs, we're back to normal," I proclaimed jovially.

On the next day I didn't know what to expect; it was my first full day home and felt a little diffident about being away from round-the-clock attention and supervision of the transplant unit. There were aches and pains in my body, especially around the surgical site and all along the incision. I was beginning to worry about the worst possibilities like early rejection or possible wound infection. My BP had gone up to 170/90 and being on the blood thinner *Coumadine*, there was a serious concern about potential complications like bleeding in the brain causing a stroke. Although I knew BP fluctuations are quite common during the first few days after a transplant, just for my own peace of mind, I called Dr. Reddy. He seemed to understand my feelings well.

"Don't worry, Ravi, this is natural. BP will fluctuate for awhile. We will have to adjust the medications a bit, that's all." He changed *Procardia* to *Norvasc*, which had a longer action, and added a second drug, *Catapres*. That worked, BP came under control and remained stable at about 148/82 afterwards.

Susheela drove me to the lab for my first set of blood tests the following day. I was eager to know what the new creatinine level would be after the travel. But at the lab, it was a mild disaster. Poor Janet, the lab technician who knew me well, became totally frazzled when she saw me in the ill-suited role of a patient, saying that she hadn't taken blood from a doctor in a while. Moreover, I was very dehydrated after several days of intense diuresis, and my veins weren't exactly popping up for easy access. To complicate matters, I was on *Coumadine* too. In the end, I wound up with a large hematoma in my left arm and neither of us was pleased. "Don't worry… you'll do fine next time. I promise to build up my veins, so next week it'll be easy," I assured her, secretly hoping to get Laverne, my favorite technician, next time.

UMMC protocol dictated that I must call the transplant center with the lab results as soon as they were available. CSA levels would be done only by UMMC and I would be informed of the results.

Depending on the changes in the lab values, the transplant coordinator would adjust my drugs as needed. I was a bit discouraged to see my creatinine level had gone up to 3.0, an unanticipated jump from the 2.7 at discharge; looked like I was on the roller coaster again! Could it be caused by the mild case of ATN after the second surgery, or was it cyclosporine toxicity?

Mary Rolfe called back and asked me to reduce the cyclosporine to 175 mg twice daily, but wanted me to repeat the level the next day. So I went to the lab the following day but seeing Janet there, I decided to go to another lab, not wishing for a repeat performance. Fortunately, the tech there got the sample easily but back came the result – creatinine, even higher at 3.3! BUN was also up at 46 and potassium was up to 5.2. Mary was sure it was probably cyclosporine toxicity and advised me to stick to the reduced dose of 175 mg twice daily for a while and see the response. Somehow, UMMC lab still hadn't processed my CSA levels sent earlier, and so I couldn't quite understand the reason for this rise in creatinine.

It was Thanksgiving, November 24, a very special day for all Americans, especially for me since I had all the reasons to be thankful for. I owed a huge debt of gratitude to many individuals. My nephrologist, my surgeon, my sister and, my wife deserved the top honors. Also, UMMC and its courteous efficient staff without whom I wouldn't have made it this far. The very thought that I had a functioning kidney now was a big boost to my morale. So many people and several institutions in the country have contributed significantly to my professional and personal success. I owed a tremendous gratitude to my adoptive country, the U.S., itself.

The Pauls were throwing a party at his house, only half a mile from ours but Susheela banned me from going, for fear of infections from the crowd. Ditto for another one the following week at Oak Hill HCA Hospital where I am on the staff. My wife was over-protective of me and I felt like a grounded kid raring to break loose!

All my friends, banned from the house until now for fear of infections, started visiting me, one by one. First, it was Dr. George Thomas and Mary from Bradenton, then Dr. Koshi and Raji from Sarasota. Others called with apologies for not visiting because of a bad cold or something; I thanked them for their consideration. The coordinator had instructed me in no uncertain terms that I had to keep myself at least six feet away from everybody. Who knew which person might be harboring what germs at any given time? All I needed was one virus entering my system in that vulnerable state.

~~~

All through the night and the following day, I was in and out of the bathroom because of the incessant urine flow that necessitated constant drinking of fluids. During a twenty-four hour period, I drank nearly six litres of fluid to keep up with the fluid loss. It was like the dog chasing its own tail. Fluid in, fluid out –truly a vicious cycle! I was determined to improve my dehydration and the overdrinking was driving my new kidney to work incessantly. Anyway, the next blood test was better. Creatinine was down to 2.7 and BUN down to 35 – a silver lining in the clouds! With adequate rehydration, the skin turgor had improved considerably. Urinary output continued to be high, but otherwise it was relatively smooth sailing. The weight went up to 141 lbs, mostly because of edema in the legs, plus my abdomen looked more like a beer belly. So I had to take some *Lasix,* a diuretic which, in turn, meant more trips to the bathroom – what a predicament!

~~~

The next day, November 27, was a much better day. Despite the relentless polyuria, I could hold my water for at least two hours at a stretch now, a substantial improvement and a good sign. For the first time, I went for a walk along the nice country roads in the neighborhood shooting the breeze and came back rejuvenated. 'Hey, I've regained my freedom, I feel okay now," I told Susheela.

I walked one mile listening to the whispering trees and chirping birds, returning the greetings of familiar joggers and walkers on the road. Looking around the garden, I noted the abundant crop of bright yellow cassia flowers, even though winter had officially arrived. What a refreshing change from Minneapolis! And I could sit down for a couple of hours in front of the computer and whip up an article for a Malayali annual souvenir magazine. Next day, two gorgeous flower arrangements from my friends Drs. Renuka and G. Ramappa and Drs. Chitra and Ravindra Nagella arrived to cheer me up. Liza and Paul dropped by with some delectable goodies and a grapefruit tree. The dark cloud of gloom gradually lifted from my mind and finally I was on the road to recovery.

30

Anemia Scare

AFTER A FEW days of rest and relaxation, I decided to venture out. My wife took me to the local library. I picked up some books, but couldn't focus well. I read the same page over and over and even fell asleep right in the middle of it. Then I would wake up with an urge to void.

At night, I couldn't sleep well; tried Benadryl which didn't work, so I had to take Ativan, a sleeping pill, to get a few hours of rest. My nights were still punctuated with several trips to the bathroom. Abdominal discomfort, probably from gastritis, for which Maalox had to be taken often, also kept me awake. Occasionally, a voracious appetite would kick in, thanks to the high dose prednisone, and I would sneak into the kitchen and forage. Watching my weight and looking out for steroid-induced diabetes became priorities. Mary had cautioned me about indiscriminate eating since the dosage of the drugs was dependent on my maintaining normal weight.

One insidious problem that cropped up at this time was anemia—low red blood cell count (RBC) and decrease in hemoglobin (Hb), the red pigment in the RBCs. This was surprising since the blood loss during surgery was insignificant. I didn't have any obvious gastrointestinal (GI) bleeding. Sometimes, the combination of prednisone and Coumadine can work havoc on the stomach, a well known fact. The test for occult blood in my stools was only trace positive.

Both Dr. Reddy and Dr. Weinstein said, "Bone marrow suppression from the anti-rejection drugs that I am taking may be the main reason." At one point, my hemoglobin dropped to 8 gm, almost half the normal and close to transfusion requirements. I was beginning to feel a little short of breath while walking.

"You don't have much more room to go," Dr. Weinstein cautioned me. "If it drops any further you may need a transfusion."

The thought of a blood transfusion filled me with trepidation, because of the associated problems, including development of antibodies in the blood that can adversely affect the transplanted kidney's health or even trigger a rejection. So I decided to wait and watch. Thankfully, the next hemoglobin was up to 8.8 gm and from then onward, it steadily went up. Dr. Paul, Dr. Reddy and I surmised that a combination of recent surgeries, Imuran-induced bone marrow suppression, and possible gastritis may all have contributed to the development of this sudden anemia. Anyway, another roadblock was temporarily overcome.

December 1, 1994

I went to bed feeling quite comfortable but around 3:00 a.m., I woke up with a pounding headache and immediately knew that my BP must be up. Yes, it was up to 166/96; so I took a 10 mg sublingual Procardia. That may have been a bad decision, my heart started pounding almost immediately. On top of that, I felt a little chest pain too. Worried, I called Dr. Raju, who said he'd meet me in the ER. My concern was possible angina or even a heart attack. If so, this certainly wasn't a good time to have that problem since I was already weakened by the surgery and its complications.

Dr. Raju was waiting for me in the ER by the time I arrived.

Fortunately, the electrocardiogram was normal with no evidence of a heart attack. With a little IV Lopressor, the heart rate and BP returned to normal and I felt better.

Next day my hemoglobin was up to 9.1 gm and creatinine, down to 2.3. My wife and I exchanged high-fives, now that the transfusion worries were temporarily over and kidney was working well. Paul joined us for the evening tea served with freshly fried banana chips. Later that night, Venu and Mini, part of my cheerleading squad, arrived from West Palm Beach.

During the next several days, life gradually resumed its normalcy. The frequency of blood tests decreased to just once a week, but the protocol still had to be observed very strictly. All test results had to be reported to the transplant center and Mary would give me a call back with drug adjustments. Once, my white cell count dropped to 2,900 and I had to back off on Imuran a little until the count came up to 4,000. By the end of January, 1995, I was doing regular exercises and eating well. The anemia was resolving quickly with the Hb up to 10.9 gm and we concluded the earlier drop had been due to the initial bone marrow suppression.

~~~

During the first week of February, 1995, I showed up at the hospital a week ahead of my official return to work – a cameo appearance. I wanted to feel the mood of the hospital staff, a test run, so to speak, being unsure about the kind of reception I'd get. Several questions popped up in my mind.

Would I be considered a sick man and looked at with sympathy or would I get an enthusiastic "welcome back" greeting?

Would my colleagues try to avoid me or would I be accepted back into their midst as before?

Would my patients come back to me or would they think, 'Who wants to see a sick doctor?'

As it turned out, my worries were misplaced. I received a hearty "welcome back" greeting from every department who knew me well—CCU, ICU, Echo and Stress lab, Medical Floors, Emergency Department, Medical Records, Personnel, Administration, and even from the cafeteria. I didn't think the cafeteria staff would note my absence. Obviously, the word gets around in a small hospital quickly. Everybody was happy that I was returning to work soon. Being too young to retire, sitting on the sidelines was not in my plans. My daughter was about to graduate from Hernando High School and I was looking forward to participating in the graduation ceremony and hearing her Valedictorian speech. Sanu had lofty ambitions of pursuing medical studies and I had to be there to support her. My son was graduating from Boston University Medical School in three months, and I wanted to escort him to the podium when he received his coveted diploma— a parent's unique privilege. I uttered a simple prayer, "Lord, please help me through this tangled web of medical challenges and keep me well enough to take care of my family."

During the next monthly executive committee meeting, I took my usual spot as the Chief of Medicine. Dr. Raju, who acted as the interim Chief of Medicine, gave the monthly report. I had to leave before 8:00 p.m. to take my *cyclosporine* on schedule. Feeling some semblance of normalcy, I plunged into work as before.

31

<center>~~~</center>

DISASTER STRIKES AGAIN!

May 23, 1995

THE TURBULENCE IN my life had abated considerably and I felt well. With my rehabilitation completed and home confinement over, I started driving short distances to friends' houses and to Tampa, forty-five miles away. I even played a set of tennis without much fatigue and started jogging too, albeit at a gentle pace. My body grew stronger and life fell into a comfortable routine. I cut back on my work in one hospital, relegating the same to my partner, Dr. Augustine, who was gracious enough to accept the extra load. There would be no more mad rush to the hospital early in the morning. My schedule was rearranged, so I could start work by 9:00 a.m. instead of 7:30 a.m. The hospital still wanted me to continue as Chief of Medicine, mostly a titular head in this suburban institution.

Susheela constantly watched over me – what I ate, when I took my medicines, when I should go to the lab for blood tests, reminding me to call for the results the following day, and more. She was always there to bolster my floundering spirit and supplement my sputtering memory, a veritable source of support and comfort. Ratnam recuperated fast at home, enjoying my mother-in-law's delectable vegetarian dishes and walking in the garden at twilight. I felt rejuvenated and reborn. All was calm for a little while.

Incredible as it may seem, disaster struck again! One night I woke up with left-sided chest pain, more like a pleuritic pain caused by inflammation of the outer lining of the lung, the pleura. Being immunosuppressed and vulnerable, I thought I was developing a respiratory infection. "Maybe the germs have finally caught up with me," was my rationalization.

It was 3:00 a.m. when the pain struck; within a few minutes, I knew this wasn't going away, so I decided to go to Oak Hill Hospital ER. After evaluation by the ER physician, Dr. Reddy's service was informed and one of the covering nephrologists on call quickly came to examine me. He couldn't find any major abnormality and a complete blood count didn't reveal much either. The chest X-ray showed minimal atelectasis or collapse with loss of air in a few segments in the lower region of the left lung. The consensus was this could be a minor respiratory infection. Since I was already on *Septra*, a good antibiotic with decent coverage against many microbes, I was sent home to rest. The pain seemed to lessen as the day progressed.

But it returned again with renewed vigor that night. I was miserable with a feeling of impending doom and needed a sedative to sleep. The following morning, I was short of breath while going up the stairs after a shower. I remember my panicked wife and sister, admonishing me for exerting myself with chest pain, but I was in denial of any major illness. How could I come down with something worse than I'd experienced so far? Also, I didn't want to miss work again. But Susheela insisted on driving me to the ER and a consultation from a pulmonologist was obtained. A repeat chest X-ray showed some new changes and the radiologist said, "The atelectasis (partial collapse of a segment of the lung) seems more pronounced now."

"Possibly a community-acquired pneumonia," said the pulmon-ologist and he suggested another oral antibiotic. All the physicians wanted to give me the best care, but none knew for sure what was happening. Interestingly, I didn't have any cough or sputum. I attributed the shortness of breath to the pain and discomfort. Dr. Acharya, Dr. Reddy's partner who examined me later, was not quite convinced that this was a simple pneumonia, if indeed it was one. He suspected there was something else going on here and his hunch proved to be right.

In view of my prior history of clots in the leg veins, Dr. Acharya ordered an emergency perfusion lung scan, which was interpreted as equivocal (inconclusive) by the radiologist. In any case, because of the complex nature of the problem, at his suggestion, Susheela decided to take me immediately to Tampa General Hospital. Dr. Weinstein, the transplant nephrologist, promptly admitted me to the transplant unit. That night, I was in continuous, unbearable pain and needed a mor-phine drip. I almost thought that I was going to exit from this world pretty soon. All my resolve broke down. The pulmonary specialist on call started me on a long-acting erythromycin called Biaxin, an excel-lent antibiotic for lung infections, but relatively contraindicated for a transplant patient on cyclosporine because of its interaction with the latter drug that will result in renal toxicity.

The next day, Dr. Modh, a pulmonary specialist and my junior colleague from Jersey City Medical Center, evaluated me. I had a spe-cial scan of the lung called V/Q (ventillation/ perfusion) scan that es-sentially showed the balance (or the ratio) between the amount of air getting to the alveoli of the lungs and the amount of blood being sent to the lungs via the pulmonary artery and its branches. A 'mismatch,' meaning normal ventilation but reduced perfusion would be sugges-tive of clots present in the pulmonary arterial branches obstructing the flow, a condition called pulmonary embolism (PE). A Doppler evalua-tion of the leg veins was done at the same time.

Voila! The Doppler study showed clots in the big veins of my right leg, and the V/Q scan of the lung scan showed the quintessential sign of pulmonary embolism—multiple, wedge-shaped defects in both lungs suggesting a shower of emboli going into my lungs for sure! Unbelievable! For the past two to three days, these clots in the legs were intermittently breaking loose and going straight into my lungs, obstructing the pulmonary arterial flow. Undetected and untreated, the condition could have been fatal. Despite hospital visits, tests, examinations by qualified, competent physicians, the condition had eluded detection. Murphy's Law at work?

Coumadine, the blood thinner, was stopped about five months after the surgery, mainly because of the anemia and gastritis. Gastric bleeding from blood thinners is a real scare. Also, a lot of doctors are reluctant to put their patients on life-long Coumadine therapy after a single episode of phlebitis in the legs or even just one bout of PE. I didn't have PE before and nobody thought the phlebitis would recur. In hindsight, stopping the blood thinner was a mistake, but who could have predicted this disastrous course of events?

Incredibly, after the first shot of intravenous heparin, a potent blood thinner, I felt the chest pain melting away and it continued to improve throughout the night. I didn't need any more morphine. Amazing what the right diagnosis and prompt treatment can do to relieve your symptoms and control the disease. The road to recovery from my umpteenth health crisis had started once again.

However, my cyclosporine levels returned as 660, a toxic level for the transplanted kidney and, as expected, my creatinine started going up, reaching 3.3 once more. This worried me since this kidney was so precious. And once Biaxin, the culprit, was stopped, creatinine came back in a couple of days to the base line levels of less than 2.0. That was a relief.

As always, Susheela slept in a lounger in the corner of my hospital room every night. With my never-ending saga of emergencies, she was so distraught and worn out to the extent that a cop pulled her off the highway as she headed home after an overnight stay with me. She had neglected to switch to the right lane when he was racing to a burglary site. She broke down and tearfully explained to him about her preoccupation regarding her husband's condition and got off with just a warning. All shaken up, Susheela almost had a mini nervous breakdown at home, yet quickly got over it and returned to my bedside with some homemade hot food. Had she reached the breaking point—I worried. I could only apologize to her for all the troubles I'd dragged her through over the years of my ill health. She was adamant about not leaving me alone in the hospital.

I was fortunate that two of my good friends, Thresiamma Jayaraj and Thankamma Mammen worked at Tampa General Hospital. Thresiamma, the head nurse in charge of the transplant unit, showered me with a lot of care and attention. Thankamma, the popular Director of Nursing Education at TGH, knew all the staff, visited me often and brought good homemade Indian food and music cassettes.

Soon I could breathe easy, with no chest pains. A week after admission, I was discharged on coumadine once the INR (a test to monitor its dosage) was found to be optimal. This meant there would be one more test added back to my monthly protocol of blood tests. Needless to say, coumadine became my lifelong companion and an integral part of the black medicine pouch I always carried with me. Now I had another thing to worry about—bleeding as a result of minor injuries, like from shaving or gardening. A repeat chest X-ray was clear; however, I would need periodic Doppler ultrasound studies of the legs to diagnose any recurrence of the venous clots.

Phew! I survived one more near-fatal emergency! However much I longed to get out of this role of a chronic patient in recurring crises, I knew I had no choice; so I resigned to my fate.

32

～

More Hospital Drama!

July 29, 1995

IN MY ENTHUSIASM to get back to my old self, I may have overdone all the "no-no" stuff like the rich food, too much time in the hot outdoors and a lot of travel within Florida to visit my friends. One evening while jogging in my neighborhood, I felt a little chest pain and tightness! Disbelief tinged with dismay pervaded my mind; could this be my heart again? Could this be an episode of angina or something more sinister? I was not expected to develop any cardiac problems now, with the BP and cholesterol being normal and I'd been doing my regular exercise routine without chest pain. I was taking so many medicines to prevent any such episodes too. Or could it be just muscle pain? But knowing my great vulnerability for cardiac problems, my thoughts went haywire. I was sure this was no ordinary pain although it subsided quickly.

Not wanting to take any chances, I quickly got home and called out for Susheela, who was working in the garden. Sandra rushed down from upstairs. Off to the ER again. On being alerted, Dr. Raju was already waiting in the ER, like an angel – deja vu! Hope springs eternal, but the EKG showed evidence of a heart attack in the back wall— 'acute inferior wall myocardial infarction,' in medical terminology! Susheela shook her head in desperation and made frantic S.O.S. calls to family members and close friends—the mini disaster drill with which she had become all too familiar.

Dr. Raju discussed his concerns with me regarding administering tPA (tissue plasminogen activator), a clot buster drug, right away. We had some fears of its bleeding potential, especially for hemorrhagic strokes, since I was already on Coumadine, the blood thinner. Dr. Paul came to the ER just then and gave me the much-needed moral boost. I was transferred to Bayonet Point Hospital for coronary angiogram and primary angioplasty, popularly known as the "balloon job." I prayerfully summoned all my Gods to be with me at this crucial time.

Dr. Raju had talked to Dr. Rao Musunuru, Chief of Cardiology at Bayonet Point. Fortunately, his partner and my good friend Dr. Zaki was available that Sunday to do an emergency angioplasty. One of the best interventional cardiologists of this area, he had done my previous angioplasty and knew me well. Since I was a complicated case, with renal transplant and already on blood thinners, my nephrologist was also informed. I saw Dr. Acharya's smiling face while I was on the cardiac catheterization table. He shook hands with me. Then I saw the face of Dr. Narendra Sastry, the cardiac surgeon, who would be standing by along with his OR crew for emergency bypass surgery if the angioplasty went awry and I crashed on the table.

Dr. Zaki was swift with his hands. He deftly threaded the cardiac catheter through the left femoral artery instead of the right one commonly used for this purpose because of the position of my transplanted kidney in the right lower abdomen and the previous venous surgery in the right groin. The culprit turned out to be a 'kissing lesion' at the junction of the posterior descending artery (PDA) that was completely occluded and a lateral branch that showed a 90% lesion. He was able to open up both arteries quickly and I was brought back to the ICU in stable condition. Seemingly, another catastrophe averted.

~~~

That night I gave more anxious moments to everybody. I was groggy with a lot of morphine on board to alleviate the chest pain. With the dye and intravenous lidocaine infusion to prevent serious heart irregularities, besides the heart attack itself, I became very nauseous, and started vomiting blood violently, the first jet out of my mouth struck poor Susheela who was standing next to my bed! This created quite a panic in the ICU. The gastroenterologist arrived soon and after examining me, diagnosed 'Mallory-Weiss Syndrome,' a mucosal tear at the junction the stomach and food pipe (esophagus) from forceful emesis.

Soon appropriate medicines were started. My blood was typed and cross-matched, and two units were kept ready just in case my stomach started pouring out more blood; however, the bleeding stopped soon. My hemoglobin dropped from 14.5 gm to only 12.5 gm, and the gastroenterologist decided that I didn't need an immediate gastroscopy. With tPA on board, my potential for bleeding was great, so I was lucky to have escaped unhurt.

After the first night's ordeal, I recovered satisfactorily and was discharged after four days. Then I went through a cardiac rehab program at Bayonet Point Hospital. Soon a treadmill was installed in front of the TV in our family room and my regular aerobic exercise resumed.

Dr. Reddy was disappointed about my recent setback. He had taken such good care of my kidneys for the past five years, meticulously steering and guiding me through the phase of transplantation and protecting the transplanted kidney with adjustment of medicines, screening tests and constant vigil. He was worried about the kidney function in view of the added stress put on the organ, especially with the dye injection.

As for me, I was glad I survived one more crisis, yet another close call. My friends suggested retirement, but that was the last thing on my mind. I decided to go back to work and maintain the status quo as long as possible. It turned out I made the right decision.

After starting work with a full schedule, everything fell in place slowly but surely. I kept my fingers crossed. Being on three blood thinning medicines now, Plavix, Coumadin and aspirin, had its own drawbacks. It's the combination of Plavix and Coumadine that wreaks havoc, spontaneous bleeding being quite common. One day I became its victim.

While chewing a snack, I bit my tongue accidentally. Although I have done this occasionally in the past without any major issues, this time, the bleeding didn't stop and I had to go to Oak Hill Hospital ER with a big hematoma on the tongue. The physician covered it with ice packs, applied pressure and gave me a Vitamin K injection to reverse the effect of Coumadin. Finally, the bleeding stopped without stitches, the latter itself being difficult since that will cause more bleeding from the tongue.

"Try not to bite your tongue, even if you have to starve, for another nine months," my cardiologist joked. "Hopefully, I might be able to stop Plavix by then."

"Maybe I can go on a liquid diet till then, so I don't have to chew or bite on anything," I said and he smiled.

Thank God, there was no further bleeding and I returned to my regular activities.

33

∼∽∼

Economic Consequences: A Medicare Dilemma

DON'T THINK THAT because I had good medical insurance, everything went smoothly when it was time to pay the bills. My travails were too numerous, so I'll mention just a few salient points here to give you the depth of my ordeal.

Before the transplant surgery in November 1994, I had a long talk with the screening medical officer of the Prudential Insurance Company, who was initially reluctant to approve the transplant procedure. However on realizing that my arguments and counterpoints were quite valid, he relented and agreed that a high serum creatinine of 7.0 with chronically progressive IgA Nephropathy would be an acceptable indication for surgery.

My sister's complete workup would be covered by the UMMC, we were assured. When both of us were discharged from UMMC, the insurance counselor came by and gave me several forms to sign along with instructions to file for a Medicare ESRD card, which would be valid only for three years; after that, my regular insurance, Prudential, would take over again.

Once back in Brooksville, I promptly went to the Social Security office in Dade City, adjacent to my hometown, to file for Medicare. The confusion with my name cropped up again (What else is new, right?). Thankfully, my Medicare card with the Social Security Number (SSN) followed by the 'T' suffix for transplantation came in the mail within three weeks. I immediately called the UMMC and gave the billing department my Medicare number, relieved that all my hospital expenses would be paid automatically now. But it turned out to be not so.

One of the first bills to arrive was from the Labs of UMMC and I promptly submitted it to Prudential. Within a few days, I got a reply explaining that the expense would be evaluated when they received the Medicare statement of payment or rejection. Many invoices from Chronimed Pharmacy, the supplier of my transplant medications, started pouring in, emphasizing that the insurance company was being billed. Soon, a second bill for $669.50 from our local laboratory for the workup done for Ratnam prior to her kidney surgery, arrived with a note that the account was past due. I sent the bill to the Transplant Center, and Mary Rolfe promised to turn it over to the accounts department. I was a little confused about which insurance company was responsible for all these payments – Prudential or Medicare?

In the first week of December, 1994, I received the main bill from UMMC, for my hospital stay, an itemized statement for $53,847.01 that ran into sixteen pages, with a note attached, "Your health insurance claim is being processed." My wife called UMMC who reassured her that the bill had been sent to Prudential. Soon two separate bills in identical amounts for cyclosporine, arrived and another bill for outpatient services. With this deluge of bills coming every day, Susheela had to get on the phone to make sure that they were filed to Medicare and not to Prudential.

For a while, no payment was being made by the insurance company but the overwhelming flow of bills was ceaseless. Prudential would say the expenses were related to end-stage kidney disease and Medicare should pay the bill. Medicare always gave us a run-around without any straight answers even after enormous waiting on the phone. Either the name was spelled incorrectly or the Medicare number was entered wrong or the suffix 'T' was omitted.

In the meantime, there were statements coming from Prudential as well. The anesthesiology group had sent their bill to Prudential, and I got the now familiar response from them, "This expense will be evaluated when we receive the Medicare statement of payment or rejection." Hernando County Lab had submitted its bill to Medicare which was also promptly denied, although the deductible had been met already.

In February, 1995, I received a nice letter from Department of Surgery Associates, headed by Dr. John Najarian which stated, "Our office will assist you in preparing and submitting your insurance regarding our (surgical) bill for your recent hospitalization and clinic visit. Please sign the enclosed Medicare and insurance authorizations and return them to us as soon as possible with the requested information so we can get this taken care of."

That was, indeed, very encouraging, and I hoped the end of this ordeal was in sight. During the past few weeks, it had been a constant battle with the insurance titans, each passing the buck as to who is the primary one while refusing to pay and citing one objection or another. Susheela, in the middle of her busy pediatric practice, office management and household duties, spent hours every day on the telephone, trying unsuccessfully to untangle this mess.

By May 1995, I was being bombarded with bills from the various departments of UMMC, including Radiology, Lab, Surgery and Anesthesia. Everybody had been notified that Medicare was the primary. Most of them re-filed the claims. On May 30, 1995, after seeing a refusal of yet another claim, I called the Medicare carrier at MetraHealth Insurance Company in Bloomington, Minnesota who referred me to Travelers' Insurance provider service. "Wait for four to six weeks. Your claim is being reprocessed," was their response. "Call another number if the claim is denied again." Helpless and furious, we didn't know what to do. Most nights we lay awake discussing solutions to this insurmountable hassle. It was absolutely frustrating, to say the least, almost as stressful as my numerous health crises.

~~~

In the meanwhile, Chronimed Pharmacy that supplied my anti-rejection medications was sending duplicate bills while waiting to hear from Medicare. On May 24, 1995, six months after the surgery, their bill to Prudential was promptly rejected with a statement "$0 of the $500 deductible has been met and this expense will be evaluated when we receive the Medicare statement of payment or rejection." I was totally surprised at this new statement since I had already met the deductible long ago! I concluded the insurance companies have a mind of their own, and I'd have to continue fighting this battle until these issues were resolved. All those-hospitals, doctors, labs and pharmacies, who gave me good service so far, definitely had to be paid. And if I had to dip into my own pocket, I was willing to do so.

On June 9, 1995, Medicare Metra Health of Minnesota informed me about approving less than half of the charges submitted by two doctors - a silver lining in the clouds at last! So I thought. However, a few days later, a long parade of bills from Tampa General Hospital related to my recent hospitalization for pulmonary embolism started arriving. The itemized bill from TGH for the eight days of my hospital stay ran into seven pages and totaled $19,794. The bills from UMMC were still unpaid, which kept gnawing at the back of my mind. Mounds of paperwork cluttered the house.

On July 20, '95, I received a shocker – a notice of 'Medicare Claim Determination' from BC/BS (Blue Cross/ Blue Shield) of Minneapolis that said: "Medicare cannot pay for the above services for the following reason," and was followed by a replica of the itemized bill from UMMC that also included $20,000 for "self-care dialysis" although I never had dialysis for even one day! No more explanations.

I was dumbfounded. After nearly eight months of intense

correspondence and haggling with all insurance companies, we were back to square one! They had summarily denied the payment for *all* my hospital bills that ran into more than $50,000! We could appeal within sixty days, the notice said. Was anybody in these billing departments paying any attention? Was everything brainlessly automated? Solving all these alarming billing puzzles proved to be truly nightmarish.

More frantic telephone conversations ensued with one representative passing it on to another, as in the game of 'Hot Potato!' from Julie to Cindy to Kevin, who demanded the Medicare benefit statements to be faxed. With additional premiums for Medicare paid, I had full coverage for all hospital and outpatient services as well as doctor's visits. Frankly, I felt lost and disgusted with this inefficient, unhelpful set up of both federal and private insurance companies. The question now was, who do I turn to that can fix this senseless, muddled mess?

I lost count of the long and unproductive calls my wife and I made to Medicare in Bloomington, Minnesota and Jacksonville, Florida on this matter throughout the past months. Many times we were rudely disconnected or lied to, regarding the existence of someone we'd just talked to, never getting the same person again, and often our calls were not returned as promised. Staring at the ceiling at night and gritting my teeth were my only options. My patients' frustrations when trying to sort out the bills after a major hospitalization now became all too obvious to me.

Teetering at the end of my rope, I contacted a Medicare trouble shooter in Jacksonville, Florida. He did look into the matter and after a few days, called back.

"What do you know!" he exclaimed like Sherlock Holmes who just solved a mystery (skipping, 'My dear Mr. Watson!') "Apparently all your claims were going to Bloomington, Indiana, for some reason instead of Bloomington, Minnesota! And that office could not figure out who you were and whether you were eligible for Medicare. I have taken care of the matter and your claims are being processed by the Minnesota office now. Let us hope everything will be rectified soon."

Unimaginably inane! Who would have thought this could happen! Nobody at the Indiana office even bothered to check on these mysterious bills. And finally, after months of hassles, on July 22, 1995, I received the most encouraging EOMB (Explanation of Medicare Benefits) from Medicare MetraHealth Insurance Co, Bloomington, Minnesota, paying 50% of a surgeon's bill. Medicare finally recognized my coverage and approved the bills. Everything was straightened out and I didn't have to dread collection notices from creditors. Amidst all these confusions, my physicians and the UMMC medical and surgical departments were very gracious and patient.

~~~

Eventually, all the bills were paid. Susheela and I let out a collective cry of joy. My health care providers were also happy, although it took many more calls and written correspondence to bring the billing and insurance reimbursement saga to a satisfactory conclusion. The total bill for this complicated transplant surgery came to more than $100,000! But it was indeed worthwhile, "All's well that ends well." Any hospitalization is expensive in the U.S. and without good insurance coverage, it can send one to the poor house. No wonder, "medical bills are considered one of the biggest causes of bankruptcy in the U.S.!" I believe our health care system needs some overhauling in order to provide every U.S. citizen, irrespective of financial status, free access to life-saving medical care.

34

FIRST ANNIVERSARY
OF MY TRANSPLANT!

November 10. 1995

THE FIRST THING I did after I got up this morning was to send a letter
of thanks to Dr. Najarian. I was so eagerly waiting for this day, a day I
thought would never arrive. I was indeed very happy. I had crossed the
much anticipated first transplant anniversary, a major hurdle for many
transplant patients.

And I know without the expertise of Dr. Najarian and the caring
service of UMMC staff and the team of physicians involved in my treatment this would not have been possible.

My BUN is down to 17 and creatinine 1.7, the best it ever has been
during the past six years. Although I have scaled down my practice a
little, I continue to work as a full time cardiologist. I am doing what little
I can for promoting awareness of transplantation and organ donation.

I constantly remind myself, the road to this anniversary has been anything but smooth. What with a major complication in the immediate post-operative period that required a difficult second surgery, recurrence of clots in the leg veins followed by an episode of pulmonary embolism, then an acute heart attack! Fortunately, emergency primary angioplasty of the block in the coronary artery corrected the latter problem and a follow up echocardiogram a few days later showed normal cardiac function.

Now, it was up to me to do everything to protect this new kidney, and I resolved that's exactly what I planned to do going forward.

35

∽

A Simple Hernia Surgery
and Its Aftermath

February, 2000

For a while, I was cruising well without any major problems. But my life must be destined to face more challenges. And the new millennium heralded itself with a new problem for me.

One major consequence of repeat surgeries in the abdomen is that the surgical site becomes weak from disruption of the muscles and the healing is primarily through scar tissue. As expected, within a couple of years after the transplant, I noted a small hernia at the site of the surgery. Hernia is a small pouch that pops up on this weak spot that allows abdominal contents to protrude into. Often such hernias do not lead to any major complication. Initially, the hernia didn't give me any trouble but gradually I started having some discomfort in the area. "Don't go for any more surgery if it all possible," cautioned Dr. Reddy, since I was so vulnerable to complications, including infections. For a while, I managed with a hernia belt. However, the hernia started getting bigger and during one of the follow up visits, Dr Reddy suggested, "The hernia is huge now. I'm concerned that if the kidney has shifted its position, it can fall into the hernial sac and get twisted around. Let us do an ultrasound and see if the kidney is okay."

Who would have imagined this would end up in a major surgery with more complications? The ultrasound images of the abdomen turned out to be quite revealing. The hernia was extensive and part of the transplanted kidney had fallen into the hernial sac where it seemed to be pulling the ureter with it! So Dr. Reddy suggested, "I think the time has come to fix this hernia. We don't want the kidney to get mangled up inside the sac. Why don't you consult Dr. Victor Bowers, the transplant surgeon, in Tampa?" Dr. Weinstein agreed with the idea.

〜〜

Dr. Bowers listened to my story, evaluated the whole situation and said, "A hernia like this can lead to future problems. The good news is that it is too big, so you won't have to worry about strangulation (non-reducible, leading to obstruction of bowel)" he joked. "But the possibility of the kidney getting pulled down and twisted around is really worrisome. We can fix it with a mesh." A date for the surgery was chosen, and I returned home.

On the scheduled date, I promptly reported to Tampa General Hospital on an empty stomach with the results of all the required blood tests. The intake counselor greeted me. After the preliminary interrogation and some checking of my records, I was tagged with the usual wrist band, gowned and then taken to the pre-op area where I was greeted by the anesthesiologist who reassured me that I should have an easy surgery. Soon I was on my way to the OR, once again.

Susheela told me the rest of the details about the surgery and recovery. When the surgeon didn't come back to the waiting room after two long hours, she had a foreboding as before. After all, the surgery was supposed to take only an hour and a half at the most. The possibility of unforeseen problems crossed her mind.

After three hours, Dr. Bowers came into the waiting room. "I am so sorry, it took much longer than anticipated," he said candidly. "There was a complication. The kidney and part of the bladder were actually in the hernial sac, and the ureter was adherent to the back of the bladder. When I was trying to separate the bladder from the tissues, the ureter got severed. I had to call Dr. Cogburn, our urologist, who repaired the ureter and that area of the bladder. He re-implanted the ureter into the bladder and placed a stent in the ureter that could come off in a week or so, which is just an office procedure at the urologist's."

Fate had dealt me a one-two punch again! Susheela and I had some difficulty in reconciling with this mishap since it was a supposedly simple surgery and that too in the best of hands. But in retrospect, I must admit, it was a complicated situation with the transplanted kidney already having lodged in the hernial sac and the lower part of my anterior abdominal wall weakened by the two previous surgeries. And there were a lot of adhesions around which the surgeon had to carefully dissect to clear the area and separate the ureter. If it wasn't done by an expert surgeon like Dr. Bowers, I guess it could have been much worse. We were very saddened, but whom can you blame but my destiny? I had no idea what this would mean for the future of my bladder function. It lengthened the hospital stay by two extra days.

A week later, Dr. Cogburn took out the intra-ureteric stent in his office after a mild sedation that made me groggy for the rest of the day. I vaguely remember Susheela feeding me some lunch at a local restaurant and kidding, "Thanks for reviving my maternal instincts. Just what I needed - a third baby to take care of!"

~~~

Once again, everything started healing well, and in a week, I was seeing patients in my clinic and taking consultations in the hospital. Something good came out of this surgery; the transplanted kidney now remained outside the sac and there would be no pull on the ureter. The kidney function remained stable. However, in about a year, the hernia recurred and gradually got bigger. After consultation with my physicians, I opted out of another surgery in that area. Already weakened by multiple surgeries, I knew that my inguinal region would always be vulnerable, no matter how well it is repaired. Why add insult to injury, foolishly hoping for a cure?

36

A STORM FROM NOWHERE!

November, 2002

FINALLY FOR TWO years now, life had been easier, without any major problems. Occasionally, I'd get bouts of upper respiratory infection, easily responding to antibiotics. I still shunned crowded public areas and took extra care to avoid catching infections. Mild attacks of gout in the left big toe and right knee bothered me intermittently, but were tolerable. I had resumed playing tennis and jogging and started attending a few social functions. But a short trip to India with Susheela was quite exhausting although uneventful, and I escaped any attacks of gastroenteritis or malaria widely prevalent in India at this time.

Back home, we went for a doctors' party one day where one of my good friends remarked how well I looked, considering all my past medical problems. The last eight years had been literally a rocky road, to say the least, with two major cardiac events – a near heart attack and a full blown one – that required angioplasties, a renal transplantation, an emergency second surgery for clots in the leg veins, a bout of bilateral pulmonary embolism, bleeding tongue, recurring generalized bruises, a complicated hernia repair, and a few attacks of flu and gout, so he was right. Just when I thought I had borne the cross for a lifetime, there came a baffling storm from nowhere.

One evening, I attended a committee meeting for our Indian physician's association in a reputable restaurant in Tampa. The chicken parmesan was delicious; Italian food was always my weakness. I drove back to Brooksville and went straight to bed, with mild abdominal distension that was written off as a result of overeating. Around 1:00 a.m., I awoke with an unusual rumbling in the belly. That was funny, since my GI tract had been one of the healthiest parts of my body so far. A trip to the *salle de bain* was uneventful.

Suddenly, I was seized with severe abdominal cramps and nausea, followed by watery diarrhea—the beginning of a nightmare that would last for ten days! The frequency of my bathroom trips rapidly increased from hourly to half hourly. Then the retching started. And soon my stomach opened up, literally. With the third bout of vomiting, there was obvious blood in the vomitus! Susheela was frantic.

"It has to be that chicken you ate!" she said as a shot of reality struck her. By 6:00 a.m., after nearly a dozen bouts of diarrhea and three episodes of bloody vomiting, I asked her to call Dr. Paul and arrange for an ICU bed for me. She drove me to Brooksville Regional ER right away.

By the time I reached the ICU, my tongue was parched, the skin wrinkled and I was exhausted. Both the gastroenterologist and nephrologist were already on the scene. Even with an IV infusion of 175 cc/hr of Lactated Ringer's solution, the dehydration refused to budge. IV *Phenergan* gave me a short reprieve from vomiting, but the tap at the bottom couldn't be shut off! Normally, my BP stayed around 130/80 with daily doses of *Norvasc* and *Lopressor,* but now the overhead monitor was reading a low BP of 108/70 indicating I may be going into a shock, brought on by loss of fluids.

My nurse, a veteran in the ICU and known to me, was almost

teary. She obviously didn't want to see her doctor in this pathetic state. With an attempted smile, she warned me gently, "Don't play the doctor now." The nurses couldn't empty the bedside commode fast enough. I had lost count of my bowel movements by now and was becoming weak and disoriented. I vaguely remember giving funny answers to the doctors' questions. Diarrhea is a dirty disease, but at the moment, I couldn't care less how dirty I looked or felt. Every inch of my body ached. Pieces of dialogues from the outside corridor filtered into my ears.

"I can't believe this! He is getting dehydrated so fast in spite of the rapid saline infusions."

"He looks toxic to me; the temp is now up to 102." "What could it be?"

"Must be a virus…came on so suddenly, right?"

"How come he has 13% bands?" (Bands are immature white blood cells and a high count usually means a bacterial infection.

I must have had at least forty loose bowel movements with terrible cramps in the first twenty-four hours of the illness. Sometimes I could feel the wild drum beat of my heart and hear the colonic aerodynamics from my belly. The leukocyte count was 9,000, up from my usual number of 6,000. Blood chemistries showed the potassium level was down to 3.1.

"We'd better move him to the transplant unit at Tampa General Hospital," suggested Dr. Reddy. "We can't handle him here. With continued vomiting, he will need IV cyclosporine and closer renal management."

So an ambulance was summoned. Susheela followed me in her car, weary and terrified.

"We're really busy today," John, the ambulance nurse, told me while loading me in a stretcher into the ambulance. "Have you been in an ambulance before?" he asked. I just nodded feebly, with flashbacks of my previous trips for unstable angina and kidney problems.

IV fluid infusion ran wide open. John's words sounded far away but were comforting. I had to somehow keep my bowels calm during the ambulance trip at 75 miles/hour with the overhead lights flashing and sirens blaring.

My new nurse was waiting for me on the transplant floor to fit me with a backless gown. Instead of using the bedpan, I braved the incessant trips to the bathroom. Soon a second IV was started. Then more blood draws for chemistries, CBC's, and blood cultures. During the next three days, my arms became pin cushions. The diarrhea abated somewhat with *Lomotil,* but I still had to take frequent bathroom trips, clinging to my wife and the IV pole.

My physicians still couldn't explain the lab results. The team of medical residents, attending physicians, nephrology and cardiac fellows, came around, often in groups, vigorously discussing and shaking their heads. I could hear some of their conversations.

"Hmm...his WBC count is now up to12,000 with seventeen percent bands."

"Potassium is still low."

"So what do you think?"

"I am worried about an invasive bacteria like E.Coli, Salmonella, or Shigella."

"We better start IV *levaquin,* especially with his immune-suppressed status."

Day two wasn't much better. Constant wiping made my whole bottom sore and inflamed. My intestines felt raw, stripped of their lining from the inflammation. Although there were initially a few bloody streaks in the toilet, these subsided, much to the relief of my gastroenterologist. I felt sore all over and was still running high fevers. By the third day, the fever abated, as did the retching and I was able to take a few sips of soup. The blood count improved, suggesting the infection was subsiding. The number of daily bathroom trips dropped significantly and the nurses felt relieved. Dr. Weinstein opined that I should be ready for discharge in a day or two.

On the fourth day, with some assistance, I was able to get up from the wheel chair into the back seat of Susheela's car. My bowels did tolerate the one hour trip back to Brooksville. After ten days from the onset of the illness, I was back to my normal self.

Later I tried to piece together all the information about this acute catastrophic illness. My physicians were divided into two camps as to the cause of the infection (if it indeed was an infection) – invasive *E. coli*, even with negative blood and stool cultures vs. Norwalk virus (Noro virus) with identical symptoms, although I had not been on a cruise ship in the recent past. (There were outbreaks of Noro virus infection in a recent Caribbean cruise ship.) My personal opinion was that I got this food poisoning from the chicken at the Italian restaurant, which must have been contaminated with some infectious organisms like a virus or bacteria or their toxins. In many eateries, the food handlers' hygiene leaves a lot to be desired, and their contaminated hands transmit the infection to the customers. Or the food could be undercooked. For most people, this wouldn't pose a problem since they have normal immunity, but a totally immunosuppressed person like me would be quite vulnerable. Once again, I came through in one piece without any setback to my kidney function thanks to the right treatment at the right time.

37

THE FICKLE FINGER OF FATE

March 2003

SINCE THE FOOD poisoning episode that ended up in hospitalization a few months earlier, I hadn't had any major brush with acute medical problems and I was beginning to feel settled and comfortable. Well, what do you know? "Not so quick," nature seemed to be saying. Wicked winds started blowing toward me once again.

One morning, a little chest tightness nagged at me as I finished my workout on the treadmill. It steadily worsened while showering. Susheela insisted that I go to the ER right away. All hell broke loose there. My chest pain intensified despite IV *Nitroglycerine* and IV analgesics. I read the writing on the wall as I started developing the telltale symptoms of a heart attack, yet again.

Dr. Raju and his partner came just in time to the ER and, after the preliminary treatment I was transferred to Bayonet Point Hospital for urgent cardiac catheterization and primary angioplasty. Of course, this meant radio opaque dye would be injected into my system and I didn't know how badly this would affect my kidney function. The possibility of my transplanted kidney failing made me shudder, but I had no choice.

I was lifted into an ambulance once more and reached Bayonet Point quickly. As I was wheeled into the cath lab, my consciousness faded. Susheela filled me in on the details later. The artery on the right side of my heart called 'right coronary artery (RCA)' had acutely occluded. Dr. Zaki, my good friend and an outstanding interventional cardiologist, who was now very familiar with all my cardiac and other medical problems, and had done my previous angioplasties, quickly came over along with his team, and opened two blockages in the RCA and placed stents there to prevent any further occlusion. The response was dramatic.

I awakened slowly and saw the faces of my anxious wife, two smiling cardiologists, a cardiac surgeon, a few of my friends, and some nurses. No chest pain!

"You're fine now," Dr. Zaki reassured me, "but you cut it too close." Later, he told me he thought he'd lost me. I'd stopped breathing, and he couldn't get the wire in fast enough. After the chest pressure began, I also had that sense of impending doom, an inexplicable sense of 'something really bad is about to happen to you,' experienced by most heart attack patients . Fortunately, the storm subsided and I made it to shore safely.

How close was my brush with death? It was indeed a close call, no doubt. The fickle finger of fate surreptitiously touched me again! In any case, I recovered completely from this heart attack and returned to work after four weeks on a lighter schedule. I scaled down the pace of life, started practicing yoga and meditation, played with our cat more often and resumed walking on a regular basis.

On my first day back (yes, I decided to go back to work since I felt good and up to it), patients greeted me with, "Doc, you have to take care of yourself. We need you." And that's exactly what I planned to do - be there for those who needed me. Although my physicians suggested retirement again, I felt healthy and comfortable to continue working. My heart attack made me realize that life, as unpredictable as it is, happens in the present. Every day now, I consciously appreciate the gift of life.

(A detailed version of this episode is included in my first book "Stories from My Heart" under "My close call, your wake up call," – CreateSpace Publications 2013).

38

⌐∿∾⌐

REACHING A MILESTONE –
RETIREMENT!

March 1, 2011

WHEN FIRST DIAGNOSED with hypertension and kidney disease in 1987, I never thought I would be able to continue my medical practice for another two decades and eventually retire on my own terms without being forced into it because of disability. Some of my colleagues didn't even live long enough to enjoy their retirement. A senior urologist in our hospital at the age of 68 was suddenly hit with a severe stroke and passed on within a few days. Three years later, an eminent cardiologist, died in his late fifties after a major abdominal surgery and its attendant complications. This sent shock waves throughout our medical community. Within the next two years, a pulmonary specialist, only fifty-four, died from a heart attack. Yet another one sadly perished when his small private plane crashed in a storm. All these created much discomfort in the community and spawned a lot of discussions among physicians.

"Who is next?" asked one doctor.

"Are we working too hard?" wondered another during our lunch hour in the doctors' lounge.

"Oh, doctors just keep chugging till they keel over," opined a third one.

Physicians, in general, are workaholics who hardly ever take time to relax. I once noted data that appeared in the newspapers suggesting the average practicing physician lives only fifty-seven years! (I know this has gone up to 70.8 as per the latest statistics). That was met with a lot of frowns in the lunchroom. Before long, we had one more shock. One of our successful oncologists was found dead in his house! Although the cause of death was not immediately clear, an acute heart attack or a serious arrhythmia followed by cardiac arrest was suspected.

A lot of rumors had circulated about me when I left for Minneapolis for my renal transplant. In spite of keeping everything confidential, this kind of unpleasant news has a way of leaking out. Before long, everybody knew about my health status and where I had gone for surgery. Even after my return to work in February 1995, two and a half months after the surgery, a few physicians and many patients were skeptical if I could stand the stress and pace of a busy cardiology practice and thought I would retire soon.

Although my physicians had advised rest for a full three months, I felt quite healthy and vibrant and was itching to get back to work after two months; besides, I had to give some relief to my good friend and partner, Dr. Jose Augustine, who had managed the practice admirably well in my absence, doing the work of two cardiologists. I comfortably settled back in my practice, making rounds in the CCU and ICU, doing nuclear stress tests, going to the OR to do permanent pacemakers and seeing a full load of patients in the office. I even resumed my educational talks for the community, organized by the area hospitals. Later, I became the editor- in- chief of the AAPI Journal (American Association of Physicians of Indian origin), a position I continued for seven years. My energy level was high, and I had clearly bounced back.

Now fast forward to 2008. My wife and I sold our Hernando Heart Clinic building to an orthopedic surgeon and moved across to the Pine Brook Regional Medical Center Office Complex, the original venue where I started my independent practice in 1984, before building my own clinic. After working for three more years, I retired on March 1, 2011.

Brooksville Regional Hospital gave me a grand send off party, a reception fit for a king, on February 22, 2011 in the large cafeteria, something unanticipated. Invitations were extended to all my patients, in addition to the entire physician community and some of my family members as well as friends. Champagne was served ad lib, and everyone had a good time. Kathy Burke, the CEO, gave me a beautiful plaque for my thirty years of service and to my utter surprise, got the county to declare the day as *Dr. Nathan's Day*, a rare honor given to those who had provided exceptional service to the county.

I was flabbergasted, to say the least. That was an unbelievably thrilling moment in my life and enormously gratifying forever. My strong spiritual beliefs as well as the unrelenting support of my loving family and friends had undoubtedly boosted my sagging morale during down times and given me enough strength to hang in there and make it this far.

April Saxer, Director of Marketing at BRH, compiled all my recent publications in the regional newspapers and national magazines, made it into an elegantly bound coffee table volume with my photo printed on the cover and displayed it at the entrance of the party hall for everybody to see. In addition, she had put together an album of all my family members with appropriate captions. There was an enlarged, poster size photo of me, displayed for all the hospital staff and my friends to autograph. Many spoke encomiastic words about me. The cafeteria cooked enough food to feed an army. Dr. Rao Musunuru, my good friend and a great cardiologist from Bayonet Point Hospital, gave a short speech. Several guests had brought retirement gifts, mostly books and pictures.

As I started driving home with my wife, I was overwhelmed by a degree of sadness. Although I still retained my privileges as a consulting physician at the hospital, I realized I wouldn't be practicing there in any sense, anymore. But I also knew that, compared to some of my friends, classmates and contemporaries who had died before celebrating their 70th birthday, I had been very lucky. Now I have plenty of time on hand and can plan for a fruitful retired life. I would take a week's rest at home, relax, read a bit and perhaps do some gardening and then decide how to focus my energy and be productive for the rest of my life. Travel was certainly high on my list, along with some writing as well.

39

〰〰〰

BEFORE YOU MAKE ANY PLANS

November 2011

A FEW WEEKS after my official retirement from cardiology practice, Susheela and I chalked out an elaborate plan for traveling to a few places in the U.S. and outside, particularly to Far East nations like Japan, Australia and New Zealand. Then in one careless moment, a freak accident disrupted those plans entirely.

While playing a leisurely game of Ping-Pong in the basement of a relative's house my right foot got caught in the wooden baseboard near the fireplace. "Was that a pop in my ankle?" I wondered, but I assured myself there was nothing a little ice and some aspirin couldn't cure. I had been in much worse situations. Probably this was just a sprained ligament. And it did seem to get better after a few hours.

The following day, we caught a flight back to Tampa. Although I was limping, I thought this would be a temporary setback, and everything should be fine soon if no stress was put on the right foot. But the pain overwhelmed me the next day and the ankle had started swelling. As we drove to the orthopedic surgeon's office, I still didn't think this was anything serious. After all, I was a fit guy who exercised regularly and did his yoga and meditation almost every day. But his verdict stunned me.

"*Raavi*, your Achilles tendon is ruptured, but could be partial," the orthopedic surgeon, also a friend of mine, stated in his southern drawl. "You'll have to wear a camp boot for a while."

"Oh my, this is pretty serious, isn't it? How does such a strong tendon like this rupture?" I asked him incredulously. My main concern was whether I would ever be able to walk without a limp. I couldn't believe this would happen just when I was ready to embark on an ambitious tour of the USA and Canada. I saw my future plans dissolving into a blur.

The surgeon went inside and brought me a pair of sample boots for demonstration. The boot looked rather big, clumsy and uncomfortable, especially since I had never worn boots except in a New York snowstorm.

"Will it heal well, so I can get back to playing tennis and jogging?" I asked.

"Oh, it will heal… may take some time, but it may not heal perfectly; you will have to take it easy for a while" he said.

"Since there is a rupture, is a surgical repair needed?" I asked hesitantly. I really didn't want any more surgery, having had my quota already filled!

"You are a high risk, *Raavi*. See the X-ray here? Pay attention to the image of the arteries, they are all calcified, even the small ones," he said, pointing out the calcified arterial walls in the ankle X-ray. I knew he was right, and it was quite disconcerting. That meant there was a lot of atherosclerosis in my body, and the wounds may not heal well, not to mention cardiac and other complications that could ensue after a major surgery under anesthesia. Being an incorrigible Peter Pan in my mind, the fact of aging had not crossed my thoughts—until now!

He sent me to Sonlife Orthotics and Prosthetics in Spring Hill to be fitted with a boot. It wasn't easy to hobble along wearing this be-hemoth with a three inch heel. "It is a good brace to restrict the ankle motion and allow the torn tendon to heal," the surgeon had advised.

For the first few days, life was rough. It looked like I was walking on pumps that ladies prance gracefully in. But having it on only one leg, the other leg became inevitably shorter, and I started feeling the strain in the left hip. So I bought a Nike that had the tallest heel.

That evening, I had to field so many calls. "What, you fell down and broke your *Achilles* while playing Ping-Pong?" My dentist and friend Dr. Ram Setlur couldn't stop laughing when he heard the story.

"Maybe I should have said tennis," I mused. "That way, I'd get more respect." After all, I have been a weekend tennis player.

My children and some of my physician friends advised: "You are not that old. If you don't have surgery, you may have difficulty in walk-ing. The ankle will become unstable, and you may fall down." One went a little further with a wink, "Hey, your tennis career would be over, so get it fixed pronto!"

"Oh, forget about tennis…I just want to be able to walk without a limp," I said wistfully. Soon a young colleague, Dr. Dan Moynihan, a sports surgeon who had relocated from New York, was consulted.

"Indeed, you have a complete rupture. See this defect here?" Dan pointed to the affected area of the Achilles tendon where I could feel a gap that corresponded to the area of rupture.

"The way I look at it, there is nothing called a partial rupture. It is like saying 'you are slightly pregnant!' All ruptures need to be surgically repaired, otherwise your ankle will be so unstable, you won't be able to walk or exercise properly," he stressed.

He reassured me that the surgery was relatively minor, and could be done under *popliteal block* (a nerve block with locally injected anes-thetic) and light general anesthesia. "Anyway, let's get an MRI (scan of the ankle) first," he suggested.

The tech at Advanced Imaging asked, "What music would you

like?" She wanted to play some songs for my benefit while I went under the huge scary magnet which always brought on my claustrophobia. I selected a Beethoven's symphony that kept my mind occupied while the loud grating sound pounded in my ears.

"Your Achilles is completely torn from the bone, see here?" Dr. Naveen Bikkasani, the radiologist, pointed out on the image displayed in the view box. The lower part of the tendon, severed from the rest, was curled up in the bottom and stuck to the heel bone, the *calcaneum*.

"So, you think it needs a repair?" I asked his opinion.

"How else will it heal if you don't fix it?" asked Naveen with a flourish of his hands. Well, it really was that obvious. Silly me, I shouldn't have even asked that question.

Later, Dr .Moynihan explained, looking at the MRI, "This was waiting to happen. Your tendons are so weak and thin. You could have stepped off the curb, and this could happen."

When I asked around, I found out that at least two of my friends had suffered from the same trauma and had to undergo surgery. Jim, ten years younger and in good health, was playing shuttlecock badminton. On jumping up to hit an overhead shot and coming down sharply, he landed on the ground with a lot of pressure, the Achilles broke and he needed surgery. Another pal tore his tendon during long distance cycling. Now it was my turn.

When I mentioned this incident to my friends, they became speechless at first, and then exclaimed, "Wow, how could this happen to you? Usually it occurs only in big-time athletes."

"Well, what do you know? I am in the company of Michael Chang and the like!" I would say with a grin. Michael Chang, one of the top tennis players in the late 80s and early 90s, also had to undergo ankle surgery to repair his torn Achilles.

～～～

I underwent the surgical repair followed by the inevitable home confinement and rehabilitation. "Absolutely no weight-bearing on the right leg for six to eight weeks," cautioned the surgeon as I left the hospital in a wheelchair, in rueful resignation to the unenviable role of a patient again.

My days got even rougher. For somebody as physically and mentally active as I was, being confined like this was quite upsetting. So, what started out as a vigorous game of ping-pong had turned into a balancing game with the walker and crutches and working with home health services or visiting nurses to accomplish even basic tasks like bathing and dressing. Depression, irritability and restlessness, followed by self-pity crept up again. Sleep was fitful for the next few days. On waking up each time with one leg encased in a plaster cast and immobilized, I wondered, "Will I ever walk again normally?"

When I sent an e-mail to some of my friends describing my anxieties and complaints, one guy, though sympathetic, gave me a pep talk, "Ravi, there is no market for sorrow. It could have been worse. So get on with your physical therapy. We want to see you walking in no time." I do believe in the power of positive thinking, but at times negative feelings just take over my psyche.

Susheela, with her superb nurturing instincts, stepped up to the plate once more, responding with great care and affection, ready to assist as needed, ever-so-accommodative and always rolling with the punches. But I didn't want her to burn out. Home health care was certainly a godsend, but still more assistance was needed. The children, both very busy physicians in the Midwest, frantically tried to arrange a private duty nurse, which I gratefully declined after my experience with an unhelpful visiting nurse who ordered me around like a drill sergeant when I needed assistance for showering and dressing.

Before returning home after the surgery, I realized that the wheelchair was not going to negotiate the steps into the house.

"A ramp would help, but how quickly can we build one?" Susheela wondered.

"No problem. I will make a temporary one for you," said Jim, my next door neighbor and a builder. In no time, he installed a nice wooden ramp in the garage which made entering and exiting the house a piece of cake.

Paul and Liza dropped by as soon as I settled in. Seeing me flail around with the walker, Paul commented, "What you need is a small, four-wheeled scooter. That will decrease the stress on your other leg, and you can get around quickly."

They borrowed one through a friend in Tampa who had purchased it for his own use after leg surgery a few months ago and donated it to his church. Life suddenly became manageable as I zipped around the house on my new scooter. Droves of friends and relatives called on us and left enough food to feed a battalion. My yoga group called often enough to cheer me and enquire if anything was needed. Even some of my acquaintances who hadn't talked to me for a while enquired about my well being. I was so impressed with the outpouring of concern and empathy. Misery became more tolerable.

After the first week, Susheela started taking me in a wheelchair for shopping and social functions. Initially getting in and out of the car wasn't easy. Soon, I became adept at propelling my wheelchair back and forth and along the aisles in Wal-Mart where we frequently shop. However, when one of my patients saw me there, I felt a little embarrassed, particularly going over the entire story again.

I learned how to brush my teeth and shave standing on one leg. My yoga experience doing balancing poses like *Vrikshasana* (Tree pose), *Natarajasana* (Dancing Shiva) and *Garudasana* (Eagle Pose) came in handy! After six weeks, the cast came off, and I was back on the boots and started walking again, only baby steps at first. The wound healing was slow. The day my boots came off, I celebrated. Walking around the garden, I smelled the roses and jasmines and watched the butterflies in motion, feeling heavenly – life's little pleasures! It took all of six months before I could start driving. "Be careful at first, no sudden stops and starts, don't strain the repair," the surgeon had warned. Finally, normal life could be resumed.

This little episode in my life taught me how important it is to safeguard your health, and how the little things you take for granted every day can disappear in an instant. In fact, it takes very little to change the entire course of your life. That is what happened to one of my friends in his early fifties. Apparently he dozed off at the wheel while coming home from his night shift and his car veered into the opposite lane for just one second; a loud bang, a head-on collision, and he spent the next month in the hospital recovering from a head injury! He had to retire from his job and go on disability after the accident. Thankfully, he didn't lose his life but for many others, even minor accidents could turn into major catastrophes. It reminds me of another friend who lost his young son when the car he was driving fell into a small ditch and the boy was thrown out of the car that caused irreversible brain damage.

The take home message for me here was that I have to be vigilant at all times. And I constantly remind myself of the many services our friends and relatives do for us in times of need.

"No more ping-pong for you!" Susheela announced. "I don't think I can take another misadventure of yours. Now that you are back to normal, I'm going to have my well-deserved nervous breakdown."

With the never-ending crises in my life over the past two and a half decades, she was pretty much worn out. She didn't even have much time left to take care of herself. Anyway, both of us decided to focus on health maintenance more intensely with regular exercise, including swimming and treadmill along with yoga, meditation, healthy diet and maybe an afternoon siesta too like the Europeans and many of our older Indian friends do.

40

<hr />

ANOTHER BOUT
OF FOOD POISONING!

Sunday, May 26, 2013

IT WAS THE final day of a national convention at a five-star hotel in Chicago. The fantastic cultural show was just over. The buffet line opened after 9:00 p.m., a bit late for my usual dinner time. While standing in line, I admired the great spread, consisting of several mouth-watering vegetarian and non-vegetarian dishes cooked by four chefs, catered by a reputable Indian restaurant and then warmed and served by the hotel staff. Two of the chefs were specially flown from Mumbai for this prestigious event. I scooped up spoonfuls from some of the dishes, including a delicious chicken curry and relished the feast, since I hadn't experienced any problems eating chicken from any restaurant lately. My wife and I returned to our son's condo late that night.

About six hours after the dinner, my belly started rumbling and getting painfully distended. Then severe vomiting, incessant watery diarrhea, and fever and chills ensued. "Oh, good heavens, is it acute food poisoning, *again*?" I wondered in dismay. The memories of the last one in Tampa came rushing back. Soon it turned out to be a major crisis, worse because it occurred in an unfamiliar city. I had to be admitted to the intensive care unit (ICU) of Rush Presbyterian Hospital by next morning in near shock. I was given several liters of fluids intravenously to correct the severe dehydration, hypotension and shock, plus IV antibiotics, steroids and more. Dozens of doctors checked me out.

During the next forty-eight hours, the frequency of my trips to the bathroom became less and less and my stomach cramps subsided. Thanks to my daughter-in-law, Sunita, an assistant professor in the Hematology/Oncology division of the hospital, I did get personal attention. The stool cultures grew *Campylobacter jejunii*, a bacterium that is often associated with undercooked poultry but can also come from raw milk and dairy products, contaminated produce or water. In my case, the chicken was most likely the culprit again! With adequate fluid replacement, antibiotics and wonderful nursing care, I recovered without any complications. The creatinine went up a bit, but returned to my baseline level within a couple of days. The nightmare ended three days later when I was discharged, weak and skinny but alive with intact kidney function. Another hurdle crossed somehow.

Later I reviewed the statistics concerning food poisoning in America, supposedly one of the cleanest countries, where cooking and serving food in restaurants and other eateries are carefully monitored. The numbers were a bit scary.

CDC (Centers for Disease Control) estimates that "Each year, roughly one in six Americans (48 million people) gets sick, 128,000 are hospitalized, and 3,000 die of food borne diseases." The pathogens involved include Campylobacter (commonly from undercooked poultry), Vibrio (which live in sea water and hence associated with contaminated raw oysters), Salmonella (often contaminating chicken),

Shigella, Listeria and E-coli from poultry or hamburgers, undercooked or left out for too long at room temperature.

Don't think fresh fruits and vegetables you buy from reputable stores or corner stands are free from contamination. We are all familiar with the Salmonella outbreak from fresh peppers imported from Mexico in 2008 and another such outbreak from Mexican cantaloupes in 2000, the green onion Hepatitis outbreak in 2003 and others from spinach or lettuce.

With the Campylobacter infection, if I hadn't received quick and proper attention, I could have ended up as another unfortunate statistic in the annals of food poisoning!

~~~

A couple of years later, I had one more exactly similar episode while visiting my daughter in Royal Oak, Michigan and my mistake? This time it was the salad from a top Italian restaurant. Once again I had to go through the whole process – being admitted to Beaumont Hospital, Royal Oak, with severe gastroenteritis and dehydration and requiring lots of IV fluids and antibiotics. Fortunately, I recovered without any complications.

Having gone through such a nightmare more than thrice (with a few non-hospitalized incidents as well), I would like to share some tips for prevention of food poisoning. CDC advises that *chicken, other meats, and shellfish should be thoroughly cooked and, unpasteurized milk and cheeses such as brie, goat cheeses etc. should be avoided.* I believe all immune-suppressed people like me are quite vulnerable to these types of afflictions and it's better to be extra cautious. Of course, when you eat home-cooked food, you hardly ever get sick, but we don't always have that luxury.

Now I am a lot more careful when eating out. For one thing, I try to avoid buffet lines in restaurants if I can since there is no guarantee when the food was prepared and how long it has been sitting exposed. And if I do go to one, I try to arrive as soon as the buffet line opens, so the food will be fresher. Often, I pile up what I like in a plate and ask them to microwave it for a couple of minutes and they oblige. Well-cooked fish has not given me any gastrointestinal upsets so far although not infrequently undercooked seafood does create problems. Salads, particularly with mayonnaise or raw egg and other cold, uncooked foods left out for a long time often harbor germs and can give you food poisoning. Fruits and vegetables have to be thoroughly cleaned before consumption. So, be careful while eating out.

41

How is my Donor, after all these years?

January 2018

You may be wondering how Ratnam, who gave me a second chance at a normal and enjoyable life is doing after she returned back to India.

Ratnam, as you know, recovered from her kidney surgery without any complications. And she was quite happy she was able to do this sacrifice for her brother. She came to USA only on August 4, 1994 and returned back to India to join her family in March 1995, three months after surgery. She got a hero's welcome at the Kochi international airport, her home town airport, where all her family members and many friends were waiting anxiously. As soon as she got out of the plane and started walking along the tarmac to the terminal, they let out a sigh of relief.

"We weren't sure what shape you would be in after this major surgery," one relative said, hinting they expected her to be a bit debilitated and perhaps sitting in a wheel chair. Since kidney donation surgery was not a common procedure and only done in special centers in India at that time, most of them were not aware that surgical risk is minimal, it doesn't shorten one's life and donors can resume their normal life style within two to four weeks after surgery.

"Oh, I am doing fine," said Ratnam confidently. "During the first week, I felt a bit overwhelmed but after that I was okay," she said confidently.

Ratnam had no problem travelling by herself all the way back to India, a trip that took nearly thirty hours. She immediately took charge of all her household duties and has continued to be active ever since. Her local physician has kept an eye on the status of her blood pressure and kidney function. She did develop mild hypertension about five years after her return but has been easily controlled with a small dose of a beta blocker drug called atenolol. This is indeed an anticipated risk of kidney donation.

We usually visit India every year and stay with Ratnam and take her around and she is always very happy to see us. In 2010, Ratnam wanted to visit USA one more time and we brought her with us and she stayed here for six months and went back. In 2012, she noted a lump in her right breast which turned out to be cancer but in the very early stage. She underwent immediate surgery followed by chemotherapy and has remained free of disease ever since. In 2016, she had a fish bone injury in her throat that necessitated surgery to remove the tiny fragment of the fish bone; she recovered satisfactorily.

At the present time Ratnam is doing well and is quite happy with her life. Since kidney disease has become quite common in India and many more centers are doing organ transplant surgery now, she acts as a local ambassador to raise the awareness for organ donation. And the prospective donors who talk to her are happy to hear the authentic experience of a real donor.

"A living donor has the ability to save a life," Ratnam says. "If more people come forward to donate one of their kidneys, we can put a big dent in the problem of kidney failure, so prevalent these days."

~~~

Ratnam is teaching everybody around her a lesson in sharing. And thanks to her generosity, her brother is living well and enjoying life fully. Because of the increasing incidence of hypertension and diabetes, kidney failure is much more prevalent now and living donors have the ability to save more lives.

42

ORGAN TRANSPLANTATION
HAS COME OF AGE

ORGAN TRANSPLANTATION HAS advanced by leaps and bounds, and in 2018, if you suffer from failure of certain organs like kidney, liver, heart, lungs, pancreas, intestines, bone marrow, etc., you can hope for full recovery with the transplant of a matching organ. Anyone, regardless of age or medical history, can sign up to be a donor. "If you are healthy and between the ages of 18 -70, you have the opportunity to save a life by giving the precious gift of an organ." Recent research has also shown that "Kidney transplants performed using organs from healthy live donors above 70 are quite safe for the donors and lifesaving for the recipients." That's welcome news indeed.

In the case of a cadaveric donor, the transplant team will determine at the time of death of the person whether donation is possible based on the health of the organ. The blood group should be matching between the donor and the recipient. However, even that difficulty can be circumvented as per the latest studies. "Patients with living donors who do not have a matching blood type can still receive a kidney transplant," according to the Johns Hopkins Comprehensive Transplant Center. Through a technique called *plasmapheresis* harmful antibodies from the blood can be removed prior to transplant. Also the availability of powerful immunosuppressive drugs has made a big impact on the whole process of transplantation and survival of the organ.

At the present time, approximately 117,000 people (all the men, women and children together) are waiting for a kidney transplant in the U.S., according to UNOS (United Network for Organ Sharing); that's the sad part. The good news is that every year the number of kidney transplants done in this country has gone up and in 2016, about 33,600 were successfully done; that's encouraging. Since there are not enough organs to go around, many would die without getting one. And a lot of potential donors may not be aware that *only one kidney is needed to live a normal, healthy life, so anybody can donate one.* My sister, 78 now, nearly 23 years after her kidney donation, remains healthy except for mild hypertension that is well controlled on a small amount of medicine. And her kidney function is quite within normal limits.

The average life span of a patient on dialysis is about seven to ten years whereas a transplant gives a lot of hope for longevity. Survival of twenty years or more after the transplant is common these days. On November 2017, I completed *twenty-three years* of transplant and my kidney function is still good. Clearly, kidney transplant is the best form of renal replacement therapy, and it has become well established as the choice of treatment for chronic renal failure. It restores your body to normal function, giving you the ability to perform well and continue a productive, active and enjoyable life.

Many are now living well into thirty to forty years, post transplant. And those who have been on dialysis before they got their transplants almost uniformly feel very happy to have come off the dialysis machine. Here is what one gentleman had to say: "Dialysis was such a difficult baby for me. So many times I had to be taken to the hospital and admitted to the intensive care unit with dizzy spells, fatigue, disorientation and low BP. I didn't know what was going to happen as my wife drove me to the dialysis center every time. Twice, my shunt got clotted and needed surgical repair. I had several bouts of infection. One thing after the other…boy, was I relieved when I got the new kidney. I am hoping to have a decent life from now on."

Much credit for discovering this new lifesaving treatment, one of the biggest landmarks in medical progress, should go to Dr. Joseph Murray who has made himself immortal by performing the first successful kidney transplant in 1954 at Peter Bent Brigham Hospital in Boston. Both the donor and recipient were identical twins, so no immunosuppressive treatment, non-existent at that time, was necessary. It's for this phenomenal achievement, first successful human organ transplant, Dr. Murray was awarded the Nobel Prize in Medicine in 1990, an honor he shared with Dr. E. Donnall Thomas, a pioneer in bone marrow transplantation.

Afterwards, Dr. John Najarian of University of Minneapolis did extensive research on immunosuppressive therapy that helped to prevent rejection of live related or unrelated donors as well as cadaveric transplants. Although he didn't win a Nobel, he has been the recipient of numerous awards and recognitions. With improved techniques and new immunosuppressive drugs, all transplant patients, irrespective of their organs being cadaveric or live related/unrelated transplants, can enjoy a long healthy life now.

Signing up for a cadaveric donor has become quite easy. The first step for the potential donor is to recognize the need and opportunity to help others suffering from terminal organ failure. Then the person can enroll in a state donor registry and also indicate on the driver's license his or her intention to be an organ donor. He or she, of course, will need to share the decision to be a donor with family members and friends. As mentioned before, currently there is still a significant shortage of available organs all over the world, especially in the U.S. And thousands die every year waiting for a donor organ that never comes through.

We do have the power to change all that.

43

MEETING WITH DR JOHN NAJARIAN A JOURNEY BACK IN TIME

Sunday, October 5, 2014

THE LONG-ANTICIPATED MOMENT finally arrived. Susheela and I took an afternoon flight to Minneapolis to visit Dr. John Najarian, my surgeon par excellence. He and I would remember the complex kidney transplant surgery on my body some twenty years ago for the rest of our lives. This was also a chance for both of us to walk down memory lane. Since a long time had elapsed after the transplant and both of us were getting older, there was some urgency to the matter.

I thought this meeting would never happen. To begin with, the UMMC Renal department secretary was understandably reluctant to give me his private telephone number. "Dr. Najarian has retired from the center, though he still retains his office here. I don't want to disturb him in his retirement. We are not allowed to give out his private number," she said. Later, she indicated that his number was listed in the directory and I could look it up. I called some of my friends in Minneapolis and local nephrologists, but none of them could get his contact information.

One day, while reviewing Dr. Najarian's work and a transplant-related You Tube interview on the internet, I came across the name Barbara Bailey, who was still Dr. Najarian's secretary at the transplant center. After some initial hesitation, she gave me his home phone number as I convinced her of my honorable intentions. After a couple of attempts, Mrs. Mignette Najarian could be reached. She was obviously thrilled.

"Oh, Dr. Najarian would be happy to see you. It's great that you called. You could come over anytime," she said amiably. "Let me know when you want to come and where we should meet."

"Perhaps all of you could meet here at Dr. Najarian's office at Phillip Wangenstein Building," said Barbara when I phoned her the next time.

Just the name, Phillip Wangenstein building, the main transplant center of the University of Minneapolis where all the offices of the specialists are located, rekindled all my old memories. "How well I know this center!" I said to myself.

So, with a lot of excitement and anticipation, we landed at Minneapolis Airport after a seven hour flight, with a stopover in Milwaukee. Rajan was there to pick us up. It was only about 7:00 p.m., but cold air greeted me upon stepping out.

"It looks like fall has bypassed Minneapolis and winter is already here!" I commented.

"Oh, we're used to this," was Rajan's answer. The drive to his house was a brief twenty minutes, and a hot dinner with red wine was waiting for us. Vatsala, ever-the-perfect hostess, had made many delicious dishes including my favorite fish fry, rice, *sambar*, *chapatis* from scratch, *chana dahl*, vegetable *thoran* and *papads*, besides yogurt and a variety of pickles. Her house was kept immaculate.

As soon as I settled down, I called Mignette. She sounded

quite enthusiastic and accommodative about our meeting the following day, and went over some details about when and where to meet.

"You can come to our place first. You know we live at East Lake Harriett Parkway, right by the side of the big lake," she said. "Then we can go to his office at the Center."

That sounded like a good idea. Later she added, "You will see a big truck parked in front of our house. We are moving into a retirement home on October 8th, so I'm glad you came before that."

"Lake Harriett is a big lake with nice scenic surroundings. I go there often to jog along the lakeside track. It's a great place to visit," Rajan commented.

Monday, October 6, 2014

After a nice breakfast, Rajan drove us to Dr. Najarian's house. It was a sprawling Tudor on a small hill with a beautiful view of Lake Harriett. Mignette was out waiting for us, with Dr. Najarian already in the back seat of the car, ready for the brief ride to the transplant center. When he saw us, he got out on wobbly legs and greeted us heartily. "You know, he has some difficulty walking after he fell a few months ago," Mignette mentioned.

Susheela and I got into the car and Mignette drove us to the UMMC Campus and valet-parked in front of Phillip Wangenstein Building. I looked at the building and premises with nostalgia, the courtyard where I waited in a wheelchair to be taken to the hotel. I recalled the busy atmosphere all around with patients being transported, and the constant traffic of doctors and visitors into and out of the building. Nothing had changed in twenty years. The center was just as busy and definitely the place to be for transplant patients.

Although Dr. Najarian had not been coming to his office on the 5th floor for some time, everybody recognized this gentle giant as soon as he stepped out of the car – from the attendants and porters all the way to senior physicians. He was most certainly an iconic figure there with all his pioneering work and accomplishments.

We went up the elevator to the 5th floor, and as he stepped out, I heard a chorus, "Good morning, Dr Najarian, it's so nice to see you again," from the staff on the floor. All the staff members were happy to see him and they came one by one to shake hands with him. His office was still kept spotless. Barbara Bailey came running to greet us as we entered the transplant office complex, perhaps the nerve center of research in Renal Transplantation in the world for the past fifty years or more.

After slowly settling in his big, cozy chair, he started elaborating on his work, memories of his pioneering studies, the obstacles he had to overcome, the reactions from his professional colleagues, and his take on organ transplantation in general. He was always ready to answer my questions. First I wanted him to go back into the 1950s, so I could get a feel of his early experiences in the field of kidney transplantation. Interestingly, even at the age of 87, his memory, especially for medical events and his research, was unfaltering. Here is how our conversation went:

Q: Tell me a little bit about your early days as a surgeon.

Dr. Najarian: I was at University of California – Berkeley, for my under-graduate studies and then went to UC San Francisco Medical school for my MD. My surgical training was at San Francisco Medical Center. That was when an opportunity opened up in UMMC. And it was a great chance to develop the program here. And Mignette is from Minneapolis, so that was a definite plus. When I came here first, the medical center was more like an amorphous complex and needed some organization.

He also talked about his ruptured appendix at age twelve that refused to heal for a long time, with pus pouring out from the open wound. And in the early 1940s there were no antibiotics, he reminded me.

About the same time he also lost his father from severe flu. It's incredible that he overcame all these obstacles to become one of the great success stories of modern times.

Q: How did you come up with the idea of transplantation as a better treatment for kidney failure?

Dr. Najarian: After the first kidney transplant was done in Brigham in Boston, I wanted to get involved with transplant surgery and further care because I knew dialysis can only do so much for the patient. Replacing the failed organ is physiologically the right thing to do. I was already a trained surgeon at that time. But I knew I also had to study immunology and, initially was looking to work with some established immunologists. Even thought of going to England to learn from Peter Medawar (the Nobel Laureate in Medicine in 1960), but that didn't materialize. So I did a fellowship in Immunology at the University of Pittsburgh and later at the Scripps Clinic, La Jolla, California, working with Joe Feldman and Frank Dixon. That gave me a real boost. It was a rarity to see a surgeon/immunologist in those days.

Q: Has the technique of transplantation changed now?

Dr. Najarian: For the recipient, not much. Generally speaking, it's not a difficult surgery. But for the donor, laparocopic (minimally invasive or keyhole) surgery is preferred. Now, robotic surgery has come into play and it has made removal of the donor organ much easier. The donor can even be discharged within 24 hours after the surgery!

Q: Did you have to face many complications when you started the transplant program?

Dr. Najarian: Technically, we didn't experience any major issues. However, after the surgery, the big question was how to reduce the immune response to the new organ. Rejection was the main problem. Anti-rejection drugs were new and there were not enough varieties. We used to give bigger doses initially in our eagerness to suppress the rejection, but ran into difficulties. Once we started reducing the dosage, we had better results. Then we continued to work to resolve the problem. And we were able to develop ALG (Antilymphocytic Globulin) ... that was a great boon. Richard Condi, our research scientist, was of great help.

Q: What does the ALG do?

Dr. Najarian: It selectively cripples the lymphocyte's ability to produce antibodies to the transplant organ and reduces the rejection potential without compromising lymphocytes' effect to fight infections. And this seems to work in the recipients.

ALG therapy is now well established as a treatment for the transplant recipients and when given early, it leads to improved immunosuppression, delays chronic rejection, lowers mortality from infective complications, and increases safety for grafts that show poor early postoperative function. ALG should be used to treat recipients of renal allografts from cadaver donors. Developing ALG was certainly one of the major contributions of Dr. Najarian and his associate, Richard Condi.

Q: How many transplants have you done so far?

Dr. Najarian: Oh, I have lost count. Many (smiling broadly), over 10,000, maybe. We do other transplants too, pancreas, liver, small bowel, islet cells (pancreas)...

About this time, Professor Connie Manskie, a medical specialist in nephrology and renal transplantation, joined us. I had specifically wanted to see her since she was the attending nephrologist who took care of me so well during my transplantation hospitalization at UMMC.

"I tried to look you up in our system. But it was difficult to retrieve your records from that far back. Nice to see you. You're looking well," she said.

We chatted for some time, and I gave her a copy of my book, 'Stories from My Heart.' She was delighted that I was doing well and was reaching the 20th anniversary. Then I popped the million dollar question: "How long can this transplant last?"

"Oh, there is no time limit…forever, maybe. Many of our original patients have crossed their fortieth year!" she said encouragingly. That was music to my ears. Dr Najarian echoed the same feeling.

Here is an excerpt from his interview given to Minnesota Medicine (MMA Magazine) some time ago on "how long an organ can function?"

"If everything is equal, and you don't lose your life because of cardiac disease or cancer or getting hit by an automobile, you are likely to live to 120, maybe 125 years. So if you take out an organ from someone who is 90 years old, it still has 30 years to go. A lot of people don't think about that. … We have transplants [organs] that are over 100 years of age."

Then he proceeded to give me his book, '*The Miracle of Kidney Transplantation*', and autographed it for me and another for my son, Sandeep, an interventional cardiologist at the University of Chicago. Dr. Najarian didn't brag about his book; he simply said, "You know, they wanted me to write about my experiences, so I just wrote it." Later, I found the book to be very well written with copious information and enjoyed reading every word of it.

After our discussions at the center, we took Mignette, Dr. Najarian and Barbara for lunch at Biaggios near the UMMC. While he and Mignette ordered lamb burgers and a soft drink, I had a tuna sandwich and Susheela, a slice of pizza. Mignette said, Dr. Najarian still had a healthy appetite. I introduced him to Marilyn, the waitress who attended our table, and she said, "Oh, I've heard the name. He is famous!"

Who doesn't know Dr. John Najarian, I asked myself. He still remains an icon and always will be, throughout the world for his celebrated accomplishments, contributions to transplantation science and service to humanity. Even at his old age, he was quite active in numerous associations and held the title of Professor of Surgery and Regents' Professor Emeritus at Fairview-University Medical Center in Minneapolis. He achieved some of the most daring breakthroughs in the field and, in my opinion, deserved a Nobel Prize. I was fortunate to be a recipient of his expertise, talent and compassion. As we said goodbye, my eyes became misty and I prayed to God to give this skilled surgeon many more years of healthy, contented life.

44

<hr/>

ORGAN PROCUREMENT
FOR MONEY AND OTHER
CONUNDRUMS

WHILE BROWSING THROUGH the newspapers at the Brooksville Main Library, a middle aged, bearded, brown-skinned gentleman approached me with a smiling face and asked: "Are you Indian?"

"Yes, of course, I am from South India," I said cordially. "My name is Dr. Nathan and yours?"

"I am Ahmed (not his real name) from Bangladesh. Came here about a year ago. I'm looking for a job," he said.

"What are your qualifications?" I gently probed.

"I have a Masters in Political Sciences from Dhaka University," he said, proudly showing me a copy of his CV.

While I was thinking of ways to introduce him to some of the influential people in the community and the institutions I know in Hernando County, he volunteered a piece of his personal information to me.

"You know, I have a new kidney,"

"Really? You mean you had a kidney transplant?" I was surprised.

"Yes, I had it almost seven years ago, in 2009, in Dhaka."

"Who was the donor?"

"Oh, the hospital there takes care of all that, they don't tell us the name…we just have to give them five lakhs of *Taka*." *Taka* is Bangladeshi currency, similar to the Indian rupee and American dollar; this amount is equal to about $6,300 in American money."

"I presume you didn't have any relatives who could give you a kidney, right?"

He gently shook his head.

"Don't they use cadaveric kidneys in Bangladesh?" I questioned.

"No way! That's illegal there," he said somewhat emphatically.

Ahmed continued to explain that in many of the countries, especially in Asia and Africa, the same rules and sentiments exist. Taking an organ from the dead body is tantamount to "mutilating the body" and is against their religious beliefs.

It seems to be the prevailing belief in several religions. I understand, in Bangladesh even the living donor has to be of Islamic faith. It's gratifying to note that recently cadaveric organ transplants were legalized in UAE (United Arab Emirates). Hopefully all countries will follow suit.

Another gentleman in his fifties, hailing from Egypt, had a similar story to tell me when I went to his gas station in my town one day. Mr. Rashid (not his real name) originally came from Cairo, but is a resident of Hernando County, Florida, now. Apparently he developed renal failure and was seeing one of the local nephrologists who recommended kidney transplantation. "But it's so expensive to do it here, since I don't have any insurance. The hospital costs will easily amount to over $75,000. So I went back to Cairo and got it done there," he said. He also didn't have a donor and through some middleman in Egypt, he got his new kidney from a live donor for a smaller amount that he somehow scraped up.

"I went from Cairo Airport straight to the hospital to have the surgery," he said.

That's efficiency at its best, I guess. I was very happy that his country could help him out by arranging such a lifesaving treatment for a fraction of a cost he would have incurred had it been done in the U.S.

The lack of enough organs to go around has created a thorny issue all over the world, especially in the USA. "Kidneys for sale" seems to have become a common practice in many countries. In India, a lot of poor people are willing to sell one of their kidneys just to put food on the table. One of my good friends in India who needed a kidney transplant, went to Chennai and the hospital there arranged for him to have a kidney that was harvested from a matching unrelated donor. They "bought" one for him for a specified amount agreed upon by both parties! Often these illiterate poor donors are rounded up by middle men (or brokers) who take a major cut of the proceeds. The going rate for a kidney in India is usually about five lakhs of rupees now (about $7,700).

I am always saddened and somewhat upset when I hear such stories of unethical practices which disturb human sensibilities. Yet in a country like India where one out of four lives in poverty, such practices like "kidney trade" are bound to occur. According to one report, "India's lack of medical regulations" and an atmosphere of "loose medical ethics" have also fueled the growth of kidney transplant surgery. The wealthy minority on dialysis can shell out enough money to buy kidneys from the poor, who are, of course, eager to supply them for cash. Can you blame them?

However, facts concerning organ sales in many countries are not that simple. While a lot of people would forgo one of their kidneys for sufficient compensation once it is impressed upon them that they need only one kidney to survive, the truth is that many unwary donors are tricked into selling their organs. There are illegal organ networking programs in many countries like India, Bangladesh and the Middle

East, where kidneys are harvested for rich clientele, many of them international recipients. For example, a kidney recipient in Italy can buy a kidney from India or Bangladesh!

Advertisements like "Kidney Wanted" or "Willing to donate a kidney for cash" appear in newspapers. Many wealthy patients from the Middle East regularly travel to Mumbai or Hyderabad in India to get their transplants and return home after successful surgery and recovery. Relatively less traumatic surgical techniques like donor key-hole (laparoscopic) surgery have made it easy to procure the organ even from a total stranger.

As Brian Resnick states in his notable article in The Atlantic (Living Cadavers: How the Poor Are Tricked into Selling Their Organs, March 2012), many are coerced into giving one of their kidneys. "After agreeing to sell their organ, if someone has a change of mind, the brokers will use high-handed techniques like hiring thugs to beat them up, sedate and drag the hapless, unwilling donor into the operating room!" Once the organ is sold, many donors feel remorseful, develop disabling symptoms and become unable to perform their regular jobs which push them further into poverty. Although the business of 'organ trade' is illegal in most countries, it continues relentlessly.

There is still considerable misunderstanding and superstition about what can happen to a healthy donor after the kidney is harvested. Most people think that once you donate, you become disabled and unhealthy! No wonder they are petrified to part with one of their organs and have negative opinions about organ donation. My own sister's friends and neighbors expected her to be very sick and disabled after the surgery. When she came back hale and hearty, they were quite astonished and relieved.

Thankfully, the atmosphere is changing now and true information that "organ donation is safe" is filtering into the lay public. More and more donors, related and unrelated, are coming forward. Periodically, I see reports of even total strangers willing to donate their kidney to a needy patient with no compensation. Nice to see altruism is alive and well. I understand the government of India has now set up a national database and transplant registry for cadaveric donation which was a taboo before for religious reasons. This is a ray of hope for patients with kidney failure there.

45

THE FUTURE:
A BIO-ARTIFICIAL KIDNEY?

CURRENTLY THERE ARE *only two viable solutions for kidney failure: Dialysis (Hemo or Peritoneal) and Kidney transplant – cadaveric or live human donor, related or unrelated. However, both these forms of renal replacement therapy come with their own difficulties, advantages and limitations. Dialysis, as already discussed before, is a lifesaving treatment, but fraught with numerous complications and poor long term survival. With regard to kidney transplanta-tion, the recipient is committed to lifelong immunosuppressive drug therapy to prevent rejection, although this is a small price to pay for getting your life back. Failure of the transplanted organs does occur periodically in addition to complications like serious infections and cancers that result from immunosuppression.*

What if there is a third alternative? In the case of end stage heart failure, Left Ventricular Assist Device (LVAD) has come into regular use now. LVAD is a battery-operated mechanical pump that helps the left ventricle, the main pumping chamber of the heart, to empty the blood into the circulation to be distributed to all the tissues in the body. LVAD keeps the patient alive with reasonably good quality of life for some time. Till recently, it was used as a temporary or stop gap therapy while waiting for heart transplantation – a bridge to transplantation – but now long-term LVADs are used as a destination therapy, which means these patients do not have to necessarily undergo cardiac transplantation.

Can the same principle be applied to create an electronic device that will simulate the dialysis machines capable of removing the toxic byproducts of body metabolism, excess water and salt to maintain normal blood pressure and electrolyte balance in the blood?

Apparently, the 'Kidney Project' National Research Team at University of California, San Francisco (UCSF), thinks so. The team led by Shuvo Roy, PhD, a bioengineer and faculty member in the Department of Bioengineering and Therapeutic Sciences, Schools of Pharmacy and Medicine, is developing (as per their website) "a surgically implantable, free-standing bioartificial kidney to perform the vast majority of the filtration, balancing, and other biological functions of the natural kidney. It is powered by the body's own blood pressure without the need for external tubes and tethers or immunosuppressant drugs."

It's too early to say if this implantable bioartificial kidney would work efficiently in most of our patients with ESRD, but certainly holds a lot of promise at this time. In the phase I trial conducted in desperately ill patients admitted to the ICU with acute renal failure, it has shown some promise. Phase II trials are now underway but may take some time before we know the final answer. Just as pacemakers and LVADs are saving the lives of cardiac patients, let us hope the artificial kidney also becomes an acceptable renal replacement therapy in the future.

46

CELEBRATING MY 20ᵀᴴ
TRANSPLANT ANNIVERSARY

November 10, 2014

AT LONG LAST, *I had arrived at that significant milestone in a transplant recipient's life, surviving twenty years after a kidney transplant—certainly a cause for celebration. It had been a tumultuous journey, from November 10, 1994 to the present.*

Can you imagine the very first surgery on my body would be a kidney transplant! Six years after the diagnosis of IgA N, I received the precious *gift of life* from my loving sister. However, it had been a rocky road for the first few years, one complication after the other, starting from the second post-operative day (as you already read in the previous chapters).

My life has been a tangled web of formidable medical challenges for over two decades after the transplant. During the ordeals before and after transplantation, there were times I thought I wouldn't make it this far. Often I was caught in a whirlpool of churning emotions. Most nights were punctuated by fitful sleep and nightmares. Recurrent psychologically traumatic events made me diffident at times. It felt like the 'cha-cha' number, two steps forward and two steps back! Wading through these deep waters to final safety wasn't easy, but strong family support and good medical treatment made me an optimistic warrior.

Potential early retirement from the profession I loved so much loomed large in front of me while going through some of these major complications. There were important family issues that gave me great concern as well, since I was the primary bread winner. My recovery from each crisis was aided by the kind attention and the best treatment by my professional colleagues. I treat a lot of patients including a few senior physicians and their wives in the community and always extend to them all the respect and courtesy they deserve. I have heard horror stories from other physicians about how badly they were treated during their hospitalizations. Medical Economics ran an article once about a physician's story that portrayed her travails after being diagnosed with cancer and how the hospital and her physicians showed an incomprehensibly casual attitude about her illness. No colleague should be treated that way. Perhaps I was very lucky to have received the best treatment available. But I know in the U.S., the treatment I got is not unique, and I'd like to think that all patients, doctors and non-doctors alike, are treated in an exemplary manner with all the courtesies they deserve.

One of my biggest thrills was to sit and listen to our daughter, Sandra's, valedictorian speech when she graduated from Hernando High at the tender age of sixteen years and nine months—seven months after my surgery. And Sandeep, our son, went on to complete his medical studies without interruption since I was able to resume my job and support his education. Susheela and I took the trip to Boston to attend his commencement ceremonies – a highlight of our lives!

Sandra finished her medical school too from University of Miami School of Medicine (UMSM), and as a doctor-father, I was allowed to step on to the dais and hand over the diploma to her, in front of a crowd of 5,000 cheering relatives, friends and faculty members. What an incredible moment! And guess who was standing next to us on the dais? None other than *Gloria Estefan,* the Latin American singing sensation, the philanthropist, humanitarian, and a great friend of the UMSM. She was the Chief Guest on that day.

Looking back, I cannot believe my luck in getting a "Preemptive Kidney Transplant" rather than one after a period of dialysis for a few months or years, at a time when the idea was not universally accepted. A recent communication from Duke University said, "A number of studies show that avoiding dialysis altogether or reducing time on dialysis to six months or less by getting an earlier transplant can benefit patients, the main bonus being less likelihood of rejection and a longer lifespan of the transplanted organ. Currently, patients with advanced kidney dysfunction are being placed on the wait-list as soon as they are ready so they can be transplanted before dialysis is needed."

My life is on a roll now. The children are very close to us and check on our welfare every day. After retirement, my wife and I have been enjoying our four beautiful grandchildren, the thrill of our lives, Anokha, 12, Kira, 7, Satyam, 5 and Sita, 3. We make frequent trips to Royal Oak, Michigan, and Chicago, Illinois, just to see them and be part of their lives. Anokha and Kira come to stay with us during their spring breaks and summer vacations. We take them to the library for story-telling sessions, book reading, magic shows and other entertainments. Trips to the petting zoo and Weeki Wachee Springs are their other favorites.

For the past fifteen years I have been doing yoga and meditation regularly; both these disciplines came to my rescue during the many post-transplant crises. Despite all the setbacks, I consider myself a walking advertisement for organ donation and transplantation. I encourage everybody to be an organ donor. Sometimes, I am asked to speak to a patient waiting for a transplant, and I comply readily. My dialysis patients cheer up when told that a transplant is right around the corner.

I am so lucky to have received the *gift of life twice*, first through an act of love by my parents, then by an act of love from my sister. And I learned never to give up hope, even when progress is painfully slow or it seems I was going backwards. There is an old Japanese saying: "If you fall seven times, try to get up eight times."

Life is so precious. So whatever it takes, I am ready to get up if I fall again.

Addendum 1

Meet the people who helped me successfully complete this most difficult medical journey in my life

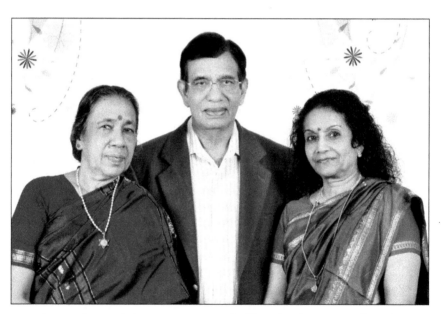

The author with his sister Ratnam (left) and wife Susheela (right)

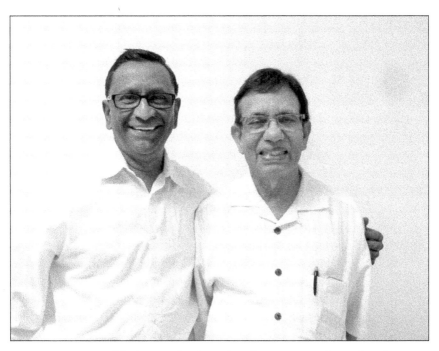

Dr: P M Reddy (my nephrologist) and M. P. R. Nathan, Florida

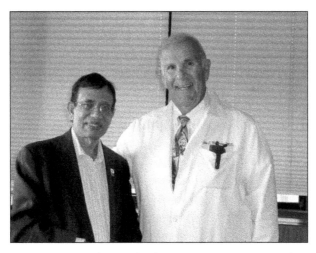

Drs: M P R Nathan and John Najarian in Minneapolis,
MN on October 6, 2014: A grateful patient meets with
his surgeon – after 21 years

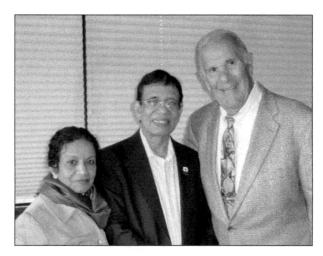

Drs: Susheela R. Nathan, M. P. R. Nathan and John
Najarian, Minneapolis

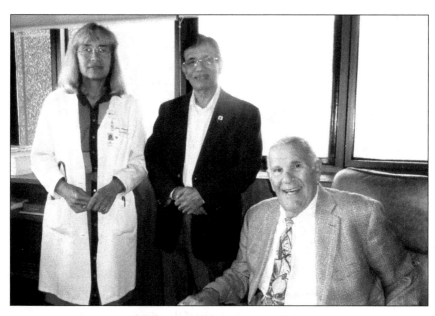

Drs. Connie Manske (Nephrologist at UMMC), M. P. R. Nathan and
John Najarian, Minneapolis

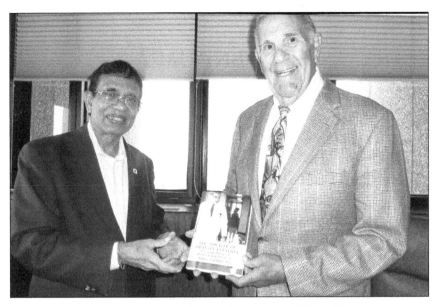

Dr. John Najarian presenting his book 'The Miracle of Renal Transplantation'
to Dr. M. P. R. Nathan

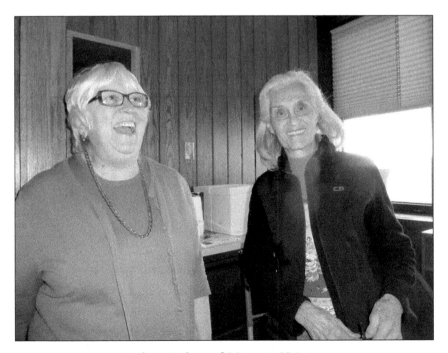

Barbara Bailey and Mignette Najarian

ADDENDUM 2

Some Tips for the Prevention of Kidney Disease

KIDNEYS HAVEN'T GOTTEN the importance they deserve in the media, compared to the heart, lungs and brain but all that's changing. With the steady increase in kidney failure globally because of the high prevalence of hypertension and type 2 Diabetes Mellitus, the public has become concerned and is looking for ways to keep their kidneys healthy. As renal function decreases and chronic kidney failure sets in, cardiovascular mortality increases three-fold. Hence, kidneys have garnered a lot more respect from physicians. When a patient is admitted to the hospital with a serious problem, we monitor the kidney function closely, a worsening renal function being a bad prognostic sign.

Many renal diseases we see in practice could be prevented or at least delayed by taking proper precautionary measures. Here are a few simple tips. Practicing them on a regular basis will go a long way in keeping your kidneys healthy.

1. Drink enough fluids

Nearly 70% of our body weight is composed of water, so water plays an important role for normal body function. Kidneys suffer when the body gets dehydrated for any reason—like diarrhea, vomiting, blood loss and even from excessive sweating.

The recommendation is to drink eight times '8-ounce glasses' or about two liters (half a gallon) of fluid per day. This is called the 8×8 rule and is easy to remember. Many health gurus think we're always on the brink of dehydration and so should sip on water constantly throughout the day even when not thirsty. Clean water is the best drink but iced tea, hot beverages and diluted juices are okay too. Beer and alcoholic beverages do not count for hydration of your body!

2. Limit your daily salt intake

Admit it, we do have a love affair with salt (sodium chloride). Most of us in the U.S. consume anything from 3.5 to 7 or 8 gm of salt every day, and in countries like India, Japan, China, and Philippines even much more. However, we need only 2- 2.5 gm of salt daily as per FDA recommendations, less for older people, only 1.5 gm (equivalent to a teaspoon) per day. Excess salt encourages water retention in the body leading to hypertension, resulting in kidney damage. Unfortunately almost everything we eat is overloaded with salt – pickles and pretzels, chips and canned products, soy sauce and salted nuts, just to mention a few. So let us reduce salt intake as much as possible. For starters, remove the salt shakers from the table and use less salt in cooking.

3. Eat a healthy diet

A diet low in saturated fats, sugar (including sugary drinks and sweets) and salt with moderate carbohydrate and adequate protein, and lots of colored vegetables and fruits would be ideal. Go easy on red meat (beef, pork, lamb etc), if you cannot stop it altogether. Shed the excess weight if you are obese or overweight and keep your BMI (Body Mass Index) within the normal range of 20 -25 (Never over 30). Nephrologists remind us a high protein diet, like the Atkin's Diet, can put a heavier load on the kidneys and can lead to some degree of cellular damage, especially in patients with diabetes, milder degrees of

CKD and those with other established risks. So try to eat a well balanced diet of whole wheat products, vegetables, fish, eggs (preferably egg white) and fruits.

Vitamin C, an antioxidant, may improve kidney function too by reducing oxidative stress on the kidneys, increasing renal blood flow and reducing inflammation of the kidneys. However too much of it, as when you take Vit. C supplements regularly, can promote formation of renal stones in predisposed individuals, as per some reports. The best option is to consume a lot of fresh fruits and vegetables that are rich in natural Vit. C.

4. Control your blood pressure

"Hypertension plays a significant role in the development of cardiovascular and renal diseases and stroke," according to the Joint National Council on Hypertension. About 25 percent of adult Americans and even more globally are living with the disease and many don't even know it. The factors that predispose to the development of hypertension include obesity, high salt intake, lack of exercise, excessive alcohol indulgence and inadequate consumption of fruits, nuts and vegetables. Modification of these factors through self education and participation in community health literacy programs will be helpful.

The recent ACC/ AHA recommendations suggest "Intensive management of systolic BP to a target of <120 mm Hg reduced rates of complications of hypertension by 30% and lowered the risk of death by almost 25% compared to the previous recommendation of a systolic BP target of <140 mm Hg. Hence, the leading heart health experts tightened the guidelines for high blood pressure.

Here are the new guidelines for us to follow. The new threshold for hypertension is a reading of 130/80 and above. Optimal BP is regarded as below 120/80. The systolic reading refers to the pressure when the heart contracts and sends blood through the arteries and diastolic pressure is measured when the heart relaxes between beats. The new guidelines eliminate the category of pre-hypertension that was considered 120 -139/ 80-89. Instead the new categories are:

a. **Elevated:** when readings are consistently ranging from 120-129 systolic and less than 80 mm Hg diastolic. People with elevated blood pressure are likely to develop high blood pressure unless steps are taken to control it. Lifestyle changes may be enough at this stage.

b. **Hypertension Stage 1;** when blood pressure is consistently ranging from 130-139 systolic or 80-89 mm Hg diastolic. Management includes lifestyle changes first followed by blood pressure medications as needed.

c. **Hypertension Stage 2:** when blood pressure is consistently ranging at levels of 140/90 mm Hg or higher and would need a combination of blood pressure medications along with lifestyle changes for good control.

d. **Hypertensive crisis:** This is when the blood pressure exceeds 180/120 and you develop symptoms suggestive of organ damage like angina, shortness of breath, change in vision, speech difficulties etc. This requires close medical attention, so contact your doctor immediately.

Please note the European Society of Cardiology and American Neurologists feel that for people over the age of 70, this criteria may be a little too strict and a systolic BP of up to 140 is acceptable in order to maintain cerebral perfusion, to ensure good blood flow in the brain.

5. Control your Diabetes Mellitus (DM):

Type 2 Diabetes Mellitus (T2 DM) is another leading cause of kidney failure. A person with uncontrolled diabetes for five to ten years may develop significant kidney damage. T2 DM has become a common disease globally, and the incidence is going up in developing countries.

Indians, African Americans, Native Americans and Hispanics are especially susceptible to the disease. In the U.S., currently 26 million suffer from the disease and about 79 million are pre-diabetic. By the year 2050 up to one in three adults in the U.S. could be diabetic, a frightening prospect. Diabetic nephropathy is well known to cause ESRD, necessitating renal replacement therapy. Use the following guidelines for Fasting Blood Sugar (FBS) for the diagnosis of T2 DM.

Normal < 100 mg/ dl
Pre-Diabetes 100 -125 mg/ dl
Diabetes > 126 / mg/ dl

Regardless of when you ate, a random blood sugar of >200 indicates diabetes. Generally the post-prandial blood sugars (60-90 minutes after a meal) should be: < 180 mg/ dl. While your glucometer gives an instantaneous blood glucose level, the HbA1c (Glycated Hemoglobin) test measures your average blood glucose level over a period of two to three months and is a better indicator of the long-term control of DM. The test measures how much glucose is attached to the oxygen-carrying protein hemoglobin inside the red blood cells and the numbers to remember are:

Normal < 5.7 %
Pre-Diabetes 5.7 % - 6.4 %
Diabetes > 6.4 %.

It is easy to keep your blood sugar under control with a combination of diabetic diet, regular exercise, stress reduction and maintenance medicines. It's important to control your urge to consume sugar and sweets. Since T2 DM affects the cardiovascular, neurological and renal systems leading to lethal complications, always pay attention to the "ABC"s of DM management – control Hb A1c, Blood Pressure and Cholesterol.

6. Control your lipids

The calorie rich, sugary, fried and fatty food that we eat daily may be killing us! Controlling the intake of your saturated fats, which in turn brings down your blood cholesterol level, is important not only to prevent heart disease but it's also important for the health of the kidneys.

Lipids or the fats that we measure in the blood consist of Total Cholesterol, Triglycerides, LDL (low density lipoproteins or bad cholesterol) and HDL (High Density Lipoproteins or good cholesterol). High levels of HDL may confer some protection from vascular disease but HDL raising therapies have not consistently yielded improvement in already established cardiovascular disease. However, high levels of all others especially total cholesterol and LDL will lead to vascular atherosclerosis. Well known to cause heart attacks and strokes, this process can also contribute to renal disease. In fact, the main renal artery can often be the site of plaque deposition, a condition called renal artery stenosis that eventually leads to hypertension and renal damage. Normal blood lipid levels are as follows:

> Total cholesterol: < 200 mg / dl
> Triglycerides: < 150 mg / dl
> Low density lipoproteins LDL: < 100 mg / dl
> High Density Lipoproteins: > 45 mg / dl

Keep your levels within these thresholds. High risk people, especially those with established vascular disease or diabetes, should aim for even lower levels like LDL < 70 and Total Cholesterol < 180. When it comes to Total Cholesterol and LDL experts believe, "the lower the bettter." The most recent studies suggest an ideal LDL for everyone is < 70. In addition to ingested fats, sugar is also an important catalyst in raising your blood lipids, so go easy on sugar including sodas and sweets.

7. Control your urge to take analgesics.

Certain analgesics (pain medications) *when taken in excess* can damage the kidneys. This is known as analgesic nephropathy. Included in this category are drugs like *aspirin, phenacetin, paracetamol* and a group of drugs called "NSAIDS" or non-steroidal anti-inflammatory drugs. The latter consists of such drugs as *ibuprofen, indomethacin, naprosyn and* COX 2 inhibitors like *celebrex.* The condition results from chronic use and abuse of these drugs. In many countries, analgesic nephropathy accounts for 10% or more of the dialysis patients.

8. Drug abuse can damage the kidneys

Your kidneys can be easily wrecked by substance abuse. Intravenous heroin or cocaine, inhalant substances like amyl nitrate, benzene and freon, MDMA, (amphetamines) also known as ecstasy, LSD (acid) and PCP (angel dust), all can lead to kidney damage. I have seen at least one young man, a heroin addict, who was brought to the emergency room after an evening of drug indulgence and partying, in acute respiratory and renal failure. Many, especially those who shoot cocaine and heroin, develop a type of "vasculitis" or inflammation of the blood vessels that curtails the blood flow to the kidneys.

9. Beware of procedures using contrast dyes

Some of the tests and procedures used for diagnosis and treatment of your illness include intravenous injections of radio-opaque iodine contrast agents, ionic and non-ionic, like *omnipaque* and *visipaque* that can worsen your kidney function if you already have early kidney disease. The level of kidney damage is often related to the amount of contrast injected. So make your physician aware of your kidney problems if you have any and consult a kidney specialist before undergoing such procedures.

There are ways to get around this by hydrating the patient well before the procedure, minimizing the amount of contrast used, sodium bicarbonate infusion to prevent acidosis and oral administration of '*N Acetylcystein (mucomyst)*,' a medicine that prevents contrast - induced renal damage. One can also do alternate tests such as MRI that will give more or less the same information but don't need contrast injection. I have seen patients going into frank kidney failure after coronary angiography using a moderate amount of contrast.

10. Periodic kidney evaluation

As part of your regular annual physical, it's good to get the renal function tests in addition to the standard screening like blood counts, lipid profile, diabetic screening etc. Your family physician will order these tests periodically but it is important for you to understand the numbers that show up on your report and their significance. The usual tests for kidney function include BUN (Blood Urea Nitrogen), Serum Creatinine (the most important one) and Urinalysis. Even a small amount of protein (albumin) in the urine is a cause for concern and will put your doctor on alert. Most insurance companies cover these basic blood tests done as part your annual preventive check-up especially if there is a history of hypertension, diabetes, obesity or any other major risk factors.

These are some of the tips that you can use to protect your kidneys. There are no specific food supplements or drugs to preserve the kidneys' health. Whatever you do to protect your heart and brain is usually good for your kidneys too.

Addendum 3

Tips to protect a transplanted kidney

ALL THAT HAS *been mentioned above to maintain your native kidney's health is applicable for the transplanted kidney too. But there are a few additional points to keep in mind to prevent complications that are specific to the transplant recipients. These include:*

1. *Always be compliant with the prescribed medications.*
   Try not to miss even a single dose of the immunosuppressant drugs and stick to the schedule and timing as the doctor ordered. Missing a dose can drop the blood level of these drugs and increase your risk for rejection of the transplant especially in the early phase. I have heard horror stories from my nephrology colleagues regarding how some patients have lost their precious transplants because of not taking the drugs properly. This can occur particularly among children if the parents, grandparents or the caretakers who are in charge of the kids neglect to give them the medicines appropriately.

2. *Watch out for infections*

Being immunosuppressed means you are vulnerable to infections – viruses, bacteria and fungus. Even a simple infection like common cold or acute bronchitis can last for several days in a transplant patient and lead to complications if not treated properly. Strict personal hygiene coupled with a good dose of common sense can help protect your body from infections. Cleaning your hands, using disinfectants as needed, avoiding crowds, and keeping a safe distance from 'possibly infected' individuals will be very helpful. Should you catch an infection, notify your doctor immediately and take prompt treatment. Beware of food poisoning especially when you eat out.

3. *Know the early signs of rejection*

It is very important to know the early signs of rejection of your precious organ, so proper treatment can be instituted without delay. They include fever, fatigue and weakness that were not present before, **pain or tenderness over the area of the transplanted kidney, increasing blood pressure that was previously well controlled, decreasing urinary output and sudden weight gain with swelling of the hand and feet.**

4. *Stay in touch with your health care team*

Don't miss any follow ups and don't be shy to ask questions and discuss your concerns. Your health care team is vital for your welfare. Get your lab tests on a regular basis as recommended and discuss the results with your doctor. Blood levels of immunosuppressant drugs are tested periodically and the dose of drugs may need adjustment.

5. *Have a good support group*

Apart from your immediate family, it is always good to have a few close friends who can give you a hand when needed.

You never know when and what kind of emergencies you may have to face after the transplant. There are also kidney transplant support groups in most major cities. Some of them are on Facebook, and you can easily connect with them.

6. *Control your concomitant diseases well*

Hypertension, Diabetes Mellitus, Dyslipidemia and Heart diseases are common in the general population and more so in transplant patients; they can take a toll on the longevity of your transplant. Keeping them under good control is very important for the optimal functioning of the transplant, your general health and longevity. Once you have survived the first few critical years and the transplant is stable, cardiovascular diseases and cancer are the bigger worries than failure of the transplant itself.

7. *Update your knowledge constantly.*

Keeping abreast of new developments – technology and drugs – in the field of transplantation is an ongoing job but you must be aware of the current advances to take advantage of them. Your transplant physician will, of course, do what is needed. At the time of my kidney transplant in 1994, I was on the drug Imuran (azathioprine) along with Cyclosporine and Prednisone, but when CellCept (mycophenolate mofetil), a better drug, became available later, Imuran was replaced with the new drug which has served me well.

8. *Avoid accidents and trauma*

As you well know, falls are very dangerous, especially if you are on blood thinners because of the risk for internal and external bleeding. They often result in surgery that will put a great stress on your transplant. One university professor I know who had a five-year-old stable kidney transplant developed a subdural hematoma after a fall that required two surgeries back to back. This led to the failure of the transplanted kidney and he had to go on hemodialysis for a couple of years before he got his second transplant.

9. *Cultivate an attitude of gratitude*

Research studies by psychologists have shown that gratitude is strongly and consistently associated with greater happiness. As per one Harvard Health Publication, "Gratitude helps people feel more positive emotions, relish good experiences, improve their health, deal with adversity, and build strong relationships." Don't you feel good when you have thanked somebody who helped you? As Louis Hay, the well known American motivational author, says, "Gratitude increases your abundance." We must always count our blessings and be thankful for them, then only we can enjoy our life to the fullest.

10. *Embrace spirituality*

Scientific proof now exists that spirituality including prayers, yoga, *pranayama* and meditation go a long way in de-stressing your life, increasing your productivity and improving your overall health. By praying to a super power, you are unloading your fears and stresses and reinforcing in your mind that you're not alone in this tough journey of life. Even if you are not religious, you can still practice spirituality.

11. *Meditate daily*

"Meditation is a conscious effort to change how the mind works," said Lord Buddha, an original proponent of this discipline. "Mindful meditation" involves focusing on the present moment without judgment and helps to keep your mind steady, strong, relaxed and peaceful. Then you can think better, act right and lessen reactivity to unpleasant situations. The tangible benefits of regular meditation include reduction of stress, improvement of emotional balance, decrease in the cellular aging process and lessening of the inflammatory processes in the body. I meditate at least fifteen minutes every morning and more if I can.

Organ transplantation has become the standard therapy for failure of many organs in the body. The significant advances in immunosuppressive therapies during the past three decades coupled with better surgical techniques have led to lower rejection rates and improved long term survival rates in kidney transplantation. A person undergoing kidney transplant today can expect a long productive and enjoyable life thanks to the pioneers like Dr. Joseph Murray and Dr. John Najarian.

Acknowledgments

I OWE A debt of gratitude to the following persons who went above and beyond the call of duty to pull me out of the many crises in my life:

Dr Susheela Ravindranathan, my wife, whose loving care, constant attention and frequent pep talks truly helped me to survive all the crises before and after surgery.

Dr P. M. Reddy, my Nephrologist, who was not only my personal physician but also a good friend and advisor during this difficult journey of a complicated kidney transplantation.

Dr. John Najarian, Director of Transplant Surgery at UMMC and my transplant surgeon, who did an outstanding job during and after surgery.

UMMC: University of Minneapolis Medical Center where I received excellent care during my transplant surgery. The Nephrology team and Transplant Surgical team were very attentive to my every need during the two difficult surgeries and stormy recovery period.

Dr. B. R. Raju, a good friend and my Cardiologist in Brooksville, who traveled with me in the ambulance during the emergency transportation to Bayonet Point Hospital during my first cardiac event and promptly attended to me during all the subsequent cardiac events.

Dr. Rao Musunuru and Dr. Khaja Zaki, Cardiologists at Bayonet Point Heart Institute, who did my first emergency coronary angioplasty with stent implant under extremely trying circumstances. They also attended to me during my subsequent episodes of cardiac crises.

Dr. Sam Weinstein, Transplant Nephrologist in Tampa, who gave me a second opinion and frequent consultations and worked closely with Dr. Reddy.

Dr. Sushama Venugopal and Dr. C. Venugopal, my sister–in–law and her husband who stayed with me during my surgery and subsequent recovery process as well as offering support and assistance on numerous occasions in the years to follow.

Mrs. Liza and Dr. P. K. Paul, our good friends and neighbors, who have always been a source of great help and support ever since we moved to Brooksville, Florida in 1981. Dr. Paul, an eminent gastroenterologist in the community, is also one of my personal physicians.

Dr. Raul De Velasco Sr, MD, Nephrologist, Miami, who did my renal biopsy successfully.

Dr. V. Nagarajan, urologist in Brooksville, who never hesitated even to come to my house whenever I needed him.

Dr. Mukesh Mehta, pulmonary specialist and Dr. Krishna Ganti, ENT specialist, who gave me excellent care during my frequent episodes of respiratory infections and sinus infections.

Dr. J. Augustine, my partner and good friend, who covered my practice during my absence and helped me in many ways.

Dr. Loretta Dawn Augustine, Dr. Niloufer Kero and Mrs Leela Raju who have always been gracious in giving moral support to my wife whenever she needed it. Dawn also gave me one unit of blood for the pre-transplant transfusion.

Dr. Showkat Kero, a good friend and colleague, who gave me one unit of blood for the pre-transplant transfusion.

Dr. M. K. Acharya and S. Hariachar, Dr. Reddy's partners also gave me considerable help while covering for Dr. Reddy.

Dr. Victor D. Bowers, who performed my hernia repair at Tampa General Hospital

Dr M. Ramachandran, a good friend and Nephrologist at West Palm Beach, who never hesitated to give me advice and second opinions when I needed.

Dr. K. V. Sundaresh, Infectious Disease specialist, New Port Richey who often gave me advice whenever I suspected possible infection.

Dr. Daniel P. Moynihan, my Orthopedic Surgeon who successfully operated on my ruptured Achilles tendon under difficult circumstances.

Brooksville Regional Hospital, Oak Hill Community Hospital and Bayonet Point Hospital that served me well during many of my critical illnesses.

Mr. M. P. Rajappan, my older brother, friend and mentor, who contacted all my relatives in India to identify the right donor and helped me in so many ways.

Miss Kim Dame of 'Hernando Today' for initial review of the manuscript.

Sandeep and Sandra, my two children, an extremely caring and cheering duo who kept me buoyant whenever I became moody and depressed. They checked in on me as needed, and helped me in any way they could. Sandeep also helped me to design the front cover and procure the figures in the book.

My numerous relatives and friends all over the world who constantly prayed for me for a successful outcome after each of my surgeries and medical crises.

References

1. The Miracle of Transplantation: The Uniiique Odyssey of a Pioneer Transplant Surgeon: By John S. Najarian, Publisher: Medallion; 1St Edition November 28, 2009

2. Kidney Disease: A Guide for Living by Walter A. Hunt, The Johns Hopkins University Press 2011

3. Transplantation 1994: Journal of Florida Medical Association, May 1994

4. NIH Web site: National Institute of Diabetes and Digestive Diseases and Kidney Disease: Nephrotic Syndrome in Adults 2017

5. 100 Questions & Answers about Liver, Heart, and Kidney Transplantation: Lahey Clinic by Hannah M. Gilligan, David M. Venesy, Fredric D. Gordon, published July 2010

6. Body Parts for Sale: Mona Charen. The Human Life Review, Vol. 26, No. 1 Winter 2000

7. Commentaries on "Body parts for sale" Tampa Tribune, Sunday, November 21, 1999

8. Living Cadavers: How the Poor Are Tricked Into Selling Their Organs: Brian Resnick, The Atlantic, , March 23, 2012

9. Take Care Of Your Kidneys: Dr. Willie Ong, Health Blog #7 – posted on Google

10. Artificial Kidney Research Advances through UCSF Collaboration: Laura Kurtzman, UCSF News Center website, November 3, 2015

11. Harvard Mental Health Letter (Harvard Health Publications): ' In praise of gratitude' - November 2011

GLOSSARY

ACC: American College of Cardiology

AHA: American Heart Association

ALG: Anti-Lymphocyte Globulin used in the treatment of acute rejection in organ transplantation

AKMG: Association of Kerala Medical Graduates in the USA and Canada

AMI: Acute Myocardial Infarction (heart attack)

ATN: Acute Tubular Necrosis, a common cause of acute kidney injury often leading to kidney failure

Abdominal Aorta: The large artery located inside the abdominal cavity, close to its back wall.

Achilles tendon: The tendon that attaches the calf muscles to the heel bone or calcaneus.

Afferent arteriole: The blood vessel bringing blood into the glomerulus

Albuminuria: Presence of albumin (protein) in the urine.

Ammayi: Aunt in Malayalam language

Anastomosis: A surgical connection between two tubular channels like arteries

Anemia: Deficiency of red blood cells or of hemoglobin in the blood, resulting in pallor and fatigue

Angina: Chest pain or pressure resulting from decreased blood flow to the heart muscle – a sign of coronary artery disease.

Angioplasty: Unblocking and dilating an occluded blood vessel, common treatment for coronary artery disease

A-V Shunt: Arterio –Venous shunt: An anastomosis between an artery and vein in the arm for better vascular access for hemodialysis

Aspiration: Accidental inhalation of food particles, liquid, vomitus etc. that can lead to 'aspiration' pneumonia

Atelectasis: Collapse of a segment or the lobe of a lung

BP: Blood Pressure

BUN: Blood Urea Nitrogen – measures the amount of urea in the blood and is a test for kidney function.

Bruce Test: Exercise Stress Test using a treadmill to evaluate coronary heart disease.

CAD: Coronary Artery Disease

CDC: Centers for Disease Control in Atlanta, GA

CKD: Chronic Kidney Disease

CT Scan: Computerized Tomographic Scan, a test by which multiple images of an organ or tissue can be obtained for detailed information

Cardiac catheterization: A special test in which a catheter is passed into the heart to evaluate cardiac function.

Cardiac event: A sudden severe cardiac condition like heart attack, unstable angina, heart failure or sudden death

Cerebral perfusion: Blood flow in the arteries of the brain

Chettan: older brother

Chitta: mother's sister, aunt

Coumadine: A blood thinner, used for clotting disorders; warfarin is the generic name

Creatinine: A breakdown product of creatinine phosphate in the muscle. Serum creatinine is a blood measurement for evaluation of renal health

Creatinine Clearance: A test that compares the creatinine in the blood and 24-hour sample of urine to evaluate kidney function… By comparing the creatinine level in urine with the creatinine level in blood, this test estimates the glomerular filtration rate (GFR) which is a measure of how well the kidneys are working, especially the kidneys' filtering units called glomeruli.

DPR: Department of Professional Regulations

Demerol: Drug used to treat pain

Diabetes Mellitus: A metabolic disease associated with high blood sugar and many complications

Dialysis: A process for removing waste and excess water from the blood in patients with kidney failure.

Ditropan: A drug that reduces bladder spasms and urinary tract.

Doppler Study: Evaluation of arterial or venous blood flow by ultrasound examination.

Dyslipidemia: Abnormal amount of cholesterol and other lipid fractions in the blood.

Dyskinetic: Inappropriate or impaired expansion of part of the ventricular wall during systole (contraction).

Ectopics: extra beats in the heart

Efferent arteriole: The blood vessel carrying blood out, away from the glomerulus

Electrolytes: Nutrients or chemicals in the body like sodium, potassium, chloride, calcium, magnesium etc. the levels of which can be measured by a simple blood test.

EKG: Electrocardiogram

Embolism: A blood clot that gets dislodged from another site like deep veins in the leg or heart and lands in pulmonary artery or cerebral artery, causing blockage.

Erythropoietin: A hormone produced by the kidney that increases the red blood cell production in the bone marrow.

FDA: U.S. Food and Drug Administration

Femoral artery: The main artery in the thigh carrying blood to the legs

EKG : ECG, Electrocardiogram
ESRD: End Stage Renal Disease

GFR: Glomerular Filteration Rate: A test to measure kidney function
Gastroscopy: Examination of the upper digestive tract (esophagus, stomach and duodenum) using a gastroscope, a flexible tube with camera and light.
Glomeruli: The convoluted tuft of capillaries inside the basic functioning unit of the kidney called nephron and acts as an efficient filter of all toxins that accumulate in the blood from our daily metabolic processes.
Glomerulopathy: A disease affecting the glomeruli – inflammatory or non-inflammatory like Ig A Nephropathy. Generally the damage to these structures affects the whole kidney bilaterally.
Granular cast: Cylindrical structures produced by the kidney and present in the urine sediment, resulting from the breakdown of protein and blood cells and a sign of structural disease of the kidneys.

Hemoglobin (Hb): The protein molecule in red blood cells that carries oxygen from the lungs and gives the blood its red color
Heparin: A blood thinner administered intravenously or subcutaneously
Hernia: A bulge formed by an organ or fatty tissue from inside the abdomen, pushing through the weakened spot in the abdominal wall (from surgery) or iguinal area.
Hyperkalemia: high potassium in the blood, a dangerous condition
Hypokinetic : decreased motion of the left ventricular wall.

IgA N: Ig A Nephropathy
INR – International Normalized Ratio, a test to evaluate the clotting effect of the blood and is used to monitor patients being treated with the blood-thinning medication warfarin (coumadin®)
IVP: Intravenous pyelogram
Ischemia: Decreased blood flow to an organ that can result in dysfunction of that organ. Ischemia to the heart muscle is the cause of heart attacks.

Inguinal hernia: A protrusion of abdominal-cavity contents – fatty tissue or intestines – through the inguinal canal at a weak spot in the abdomen.

IVP: Intravenous Pyelogram, a radiological procedure that uses intravenous contrast to detect abnormalities in the kidney, ureter or bladder.

Immunology: Study of the immune system in the body

Kuchipudi: A form of Indian classical dance that originated in a village named Kuchipudi in the Indian state of Andhra Pradesh

LRD: Living related donor

Lopressor: A beta blocker that reduces the heart rate and improves the blood pressure

LV: Left ventricle

MRI: Magnetic Resonance Imaging: A test that uses magnetic field to image the organs inside the body

Mallory – Weiss Syndrome: A tear in the mucosa of the lower esophagus that can bleed, often caused by prolonged and violent vomiting.

Medicare: Medical Insurance Plan administered by the Federal Government

Mucomyst: N Acetylcystine, a drug that protects the kidneys during contrast imaging during angiogram. Myocardial Ischemia: Decreased blood flow to the heart muscle that can result in heart attacks.

Myocardial Infarction: A heart attack usually from blockage of a coronary artery

NPO: Nothing by mouth

Nephrologist: A doctor specializing in kidney diseases

Nephropathy: A general term suggesting disease of, or damage to the kidneys

Nephrectomy: Surgical removal of a kidney

Occult blood in the stools: Presence of blood not visibly apparent but can be detected through special test.

OR: Operating room

Oxalosis: A rare metabolic disorder in which the kidneys are unable to excrete calcium oxalate from the body

PE: Pulmonary embolism, clots in the lungs

PRO: Peer Review Organization

Perfusion scan: A special scan of the lungs to detect clots – pulmonary embolism

Plasmapheresis: A blood purification procedure in which harmful antibodies from the plasma is first removed to limit the rejection process when a "kidney transplant is done from a blood type incompatible donor."

Pleura: the outer covering of the lungs.

Pleuritic: relating to pleura or outer covering of the lungs. Pleurisy is inflammation of the pleura.

Post-Prandial: After meals

Polyuria: Abnormally large production or passage of dilute urine, urinary output exceeding 2.5 – 3 Liters / day

Prudential: A medical and life insurance company

Pulmonary embolism: Clots blocking one or more of the pulmonary arteries in the lungs that travel from the legs.

Pulmonologist: A specialist in lung diseases

Rejection: Loss of function of kidney transplant because the body may recognize the transplanted organ as a foreign object

Renal replacement therapy: Therapy that replaces renal function and includes hemodialysis, peritoneal dialysis, blood purification and renal transplantation.

Sari: A long garment draped around the body by females in India

Strangulation of hernia: The contents of the hernia becoming trapped at the weak point in the abdominal wall leading to obstruction of the bowel, a serious condition.

Subdural Hematoma: A collection of blood below the inner covering of the brain called dura but outside the brain and usually results from severe head trauma.

tPA: Tissue plasminogen activator, a drug that dissolves the clot in an artery.

TGH: Tampa General Hospital, Tampa

UMMC: University of Minneapolis Medical Center, Minneapolis, MN

Ureter: the duct (tube) that carries urine from the kidneys to the bladder

VQ Scan: Ventillation Perfusion scan, a nuclear scan that examines both the airflow and blood flow in the lungs and generally thought to be specific for the diagnosis of pulmonary embolism.

Venous thrombosis: clots in the veins - commonly occurring in the leg veins

Vrikshasana, Natarajasana, Garudasana: The original Sanskrit names for the various Yoga postures

Praise for **Second Chance**

A compelling, multi-faceted, richly textured, meticulous account of a kidney transplant by a noted physician, offering deeply personal and highly professional insights, informed by compassion and passion. A significant original contribution to the literature on kidney transplantation.

> *Dr. Chennat Gopalakrishnan*
> Professor Emeritus, University of Hawaii at Manoa
> Editor-in-Chief, Journal of Natural Resources
> Policy Research

The renowned cardiologist Dr. M P Ravindra Nathan who had treated thousands of patients for quarter of a century, took an unexpected turn to be on the other end of the stethoscope as a patient in kidney failure, and received a live kidney transplant from his loving sister who came all the way from India to give him the new gift of life.

After continuing in active medical practice for another quarter of a century with the transplanted kidney, Dr. Nathan in this book gives an insider's peek into his daunting, but courageous journey with the new kidney. It is a very touching and inspiring human story of extraordinary courage, but it is also an excellent reassuring guide for all facing life-threatening illnesses, especially to those thinking of receiving a kidney transplant, or to those planning to donate one of their kidneys as a live donor.

> *Roy P Thomas, MD*
> Physician (Internist), trained in India, England and U.S Writer, Speaker, and has been hosting a weekly medical program on Kairali TV, Kerala, India for the past 14 years.

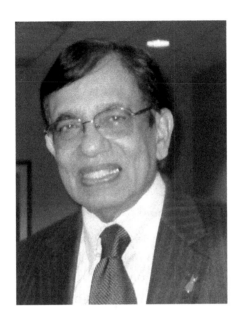

***Dr. M. P. Ravindra Nathan MBBS, FACC, FACP, FRCP (Lond),
FRCP (C), FAHA*** is a physician with over fifty years of experience in
the practice of medicine and cardiology. He was the Associate Director
of Cardiology at Jersey City Medical Center, NJ and Clinical Asst.
Professor of Medicine at New Jersey College of Medicine, Newark,
N.J. He moved to Florida in 1981 for cardiovascular practice and established Hernando Heart Clinic in Brooksville, Florida in 1987 and
worked as its director for 21 years. Currently, he is retired but works
as a volunteer cardiologist at the Crescent Community Free Clinic,
Spring Hill, Florida. He is also an author, speaker, and a humanitarian.

Dr. Nathan was born in India and received his MBBS (equivalent
to MD in USA) from Trivandrum Medical College, India, where he received a full scholarship during his medical studies. He then completed

his post-graduate medical training in England working in different hospitals in London, Cambridge, Sheffield, and Sunderland and received the much-coveted degree of MRCP (London). He came to the United States in 1972 with his wife, Dr. Susheela.

Dr. Nathan is board certified in Internal medicine as well as Cardiovascular diseases and is a Fellow of the Royal College of Physicians of London (FRCP), Royal College of Physicians of Canada (FRCP – C), American College of Physicians (FACP), American College of Cardiology (FACC) and American Heart Association (FAHA).

He is also a founding member and the past president of AKMG (Association of Kerala Medical Graduates) and a past president of the Hernando Medical Society and Hernando division of the American Heart Association.

He has published over 200 articles and stories including research papers in scientific journals and lay press. Dr. Nathan has been a frequent contributor to *Medical Economics, Cortlandt Forum, Journal of the Florida Medical Association, Tampa Bay Times*, and *Hernando Today*, and writes a monthly column on medical matters for *Khaas Baat*, an Indian newsmagazine. He was the Editor-in-Chief of the *AAPI Journal* for many years and is currently its Emeritus Editor. Dr. Nathan edited, along with five co-authors, a coffee table volume of 215 pages titled *Archives of AKMG*, which was released on July 13, 2012 in Detroit by the President of American Medical Association, Dr. Jeremy Lazarus.

Dr. Nathan released his first book, "Stories from My Heart – *A Cardiologist's Reflections on the Gift of Life*" in 2013.

CPSIA information can be obtained
at www.ICGtesting.com
Printed in the USA
BVHW040202301019
562462BV00002B/3/P